# Complications in Laparoscopic Surgery

Cavit Avci • José M. Schiappa

Editors

# Complications in Laparoscopic Surgery

## A Guide to Prevention and Management

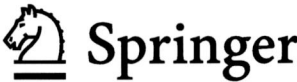 Springer

*Editors*
Cavit Avci
General and Laparoscopic Surgery
Istanbul University Medical School
Istanbul
Turkey

José M. Schiappa
Department of Surgery
Hospital CUF Infante Santo
Lisbon
Portugal

ISBN 978-3-319-19622-0      ISBN 978-3-319-19623-7   (eBook)
DOI 10.1007/978-3-319-19623-7

Library of Congress Control Number: 2015954103

Springer Cham Heidelberg New York Dordrecht London

Printed on acid-free paper

Springer International Publishing AG Switzerland is part of Springer Science+Business Media
(www.springer.com)

# Foreword

Not willing to prejudge what professional historians will decide, those in charge of writing history with a capital "H," the starting point of the endo-laparoscopic revolution in digestive surgery can be pinpointed to around 1987, the dawn of the last decade of the twentieth century. In 2015, the middle of the second decade of the twenty-first century, the maturation of results already validated allows for a constructive critical inventory. This shows how timely the book conceived and realized by José Schiappa and Cavit Avci, and by the expert contributors they have invited, is. Receiving their invitation to write this preface was a great honor for me and I am grateful to them for it. They also gave me the pleasure of being the first person to read the book, and I have no doubt that future readers will be equally delighted.

*The title* gives clues: *Complications in Laparoscopic Surgery. A Guidebook to Prevention and Management.* Is it possible that a quarter century after its beginning, the new way to perform surgery, so contested in the beginning and having finally spread all over the planet, can still cause complications? The answer is "Yes," because errors are still possible in choosing appropriate indications, and gaps still persist in some teaching programs devoted to good technical practice. We must congratulate the authors for having the courage to recognize these aspects and to try to find a solution for correcting them; this is imperative for reinforcing our patients' safety and satisfaction. Nowadays, medical literature is more focused on "novelties and advanced techniques" – options that can indeed seem more attractive to younger generations, but are too recent to be considered definitively validated. It is premature to make a proper choice between marketing announcements without a future and beginnings of promising developments that are possibly sustainable; let these novelties first cross the "filter" of scientific studies done by reliable, specialized institutions.

Let us focus our attention on this book's enhancing the relevance of everyday laparoscopic surgery, renamed "*conventional* laparoscopic surgery" after 25 years of uninterrupted successes. In this way we can teach it better and fine-tune it. We can consolidate what is already the trustworthy platform for launching new techniques in the clinical testing phase and also the trusted refuge in case of the test's failure – in which case the surgeon can always return to a conventional validated laparoscopic procedure during the same surgery, a true guarantee for the patient's safety. This has been our *golden rule* since 1989, when we launched the first procedures of endo-laparoscopic surgery. At that time, the only option was reverting to open surgery. For the time being, that *golden rule* must remain our priority, but the surgeon now has the choice of returning to other options that are already within the realm of conventional endo-laparoscopic procedures that are so beneficial for our patients.

*"Efficient surgery combined with patients' safety"* is the goal of this book; to reach that goal, I invite you to read it attentively.

*There are* seven chapters, each one having been selected by the editors to provide an example of the seriousness of their experiences, described from the point of view of complications.

Chapter 1. It is not possible to perform any laparoscopic surgery without first creating a space to work in under the closed abdominal wall of the patient. This is a subject of general interest regarding the establishment of the pneumoperitoneum by insufflating the abdominal cavity (also called the "coelomic cavity"). The reason that the term "coelio-surgery" [1] is preferred is that it is more precise – at least in the French language – than laparoscopic surgery. Insufflation of the virtual cavity needs very precise maneuvers and a complete respect for the safety tests in order to avoid serious or even lethal complications, and recent statistics have confirmed this. Levent Avtan, the author of this chapter, gives a complete review of how to program minimally invasive surgery so it does not turn into tragedy.

Chapters 2, 3, 4, 5, 6, and 7 address global issues, with some observations about the history of surgery (especially Chaps. 2 and 3). Each chapter is devoted to a particular procedure that was chosen because it had been scientifically confirmed for a long time and is performed daily all over the world. Each of the authors presents his own personal concept of the intervention he writes about, describing their indications, their technical techniques, an exhaustive description of all possible complications and their causes, ways of treatment, and ways of prevention while always trying to maintain, as much as possible, the advantages for the patient of the minimally invasive approach. They describe their strategies, their own prescriptions, advice, and "tips and tricks" in order to avoid any pitfalls that might be hidden, even at the early stage of choosing the right operative procedure, as well as at the second stage, i.e., during the chosen procedure's progression.

Although the authors have written the chapters based on their own personal experiences, reading them gives the impression of a great homogeneity of points of view. This confirms the concept of the uniqueness of surgery that we considered as fundamental since the very beginnings of minimally invasive surgery. We were "hammering out" that principle in France during the early conferences, and to our first visitors, with Philippe Mouret, François Dubois, Edmond Estour, Pierre Testas, François Drouard, and also with our first assistants, who soon became our first emulators between 1987 and 1989. "Let's not oppose open surgery to endo-laparoscopic surgery. The latter is a divergent branch merging from the central trunk of evolution of open surgery, as a result of oncoming technical innovations. We have to integrate them at the right places for the greater patients' benefits. This does not mean the disappearance of open surgery; on the contrary, it will continue its own evolution with its own indications and its further merging of new innovative branches." This concept was to us non-questionable evidence, as it matches the patients' endless demand "to be treated at best with the fewest possible adverse side effects." Endoscopy opened for them the era of more comfortable surgery – the minimally invasive surgery whose limits of expansion are not yet determinable today.

Between 1987 and 1990, the only visceral surgeons with this point of view were the gynecologists [2], who took the great step forward in 1973, moving from exploratory laparoscopy to surgical laparoscopy to cure ectopic pregnancy. We were very few then, with the digestive tract surgeons following closely this evolution; the reason was that around 1975, with the beginning of the creation of separate medical specialities, the module dedicated to gynecologic procedures became optional in the educational program for residents in general surgery, and few people made that choice, which was completely abandoned later on. In 1988, very few digestive surgeons were able to understand how the invention of the minivideocamera made surgery possible without laparotomy. The great majority of them were fascinated by the dazzling successes of open surgery, then at the apogee of its development. In addition, the professors in charge of their education taught them that the unavoidable price to pay for these successes was the drawbacks of laparotomy. The larger they are, the more they allow better intra-corporeal vision and a deeper penetration of the surgeon's hands in reaching the operating field. "For big surgeons, big incisions" was the popular saying. Our small group of "pro-coelioscopists" thought exactly the opposite, that there was no need to open in order to see better, and the duo of laparoscope and minivideocameras will take care of that, making the introduction of hands deep inside a patient's body unnecessary. Surgeons' hands will work from a distance, outside the body, maneuvering more and more sophisticated tools.

From the start, we were absolutely certainty that we had the key to the future of surgery, but first we had to convince others. The operative handling of laparoscopy was different from that of open surgery and learning it necessitated a long and difficult training period with, at that time, very basic tools that did not allow for complex maneuvers. All this made its practice difficult and potentially dangerous for a small number of indications. Beginning in 1988, the minivideocamera worked as our "absolute convincing weapon" for that purpose, especially when it became easier to purchase. It was quite good at changing the minds of the "coelio-indifferent" and "coelio-skeptical;" fortunately, the latter were more numerous. In fact, it was not as successful among the "anti-laparoscopy-by-principle" adherents. They were not numerous, but they were important as their group included almost all the main leaders of academic teachers in digestive surgery. The solution was to subtly introduce our "absolute weapon" inside the scientific societies in charge of validating research and teaching works concerning therapeutic innovations. This type of society already existed in Europe (Germany, Benelux, France, Italy), but they usually worked without real interconnections, having a weak impact regarding innovations in surgical procedures. We managed to unify them and make them more efficient, by founding, for instance, EAES [3] in 1989–1990, after receiving advice from our American colleagues. In 1981 in the U.S., they founded SAGES [4], a society that had as its objective the creation of a program of education and research in endoscopic endolumenal digestive surgery, conceived by surgeons for surgeons and obtaining its accreditation from the federal authorities in charge of these matters, which was achieved around 1986. For the founders of EAES, it was the best model to follow.

In Europe, despite free access to our operating rooms, which were open to all surgeons who wanted to visit, the use of our "absolute weapon" in live demonstration sessions during our first symposia, the progress remained rather modest regarding the acceptance of this new kind of surgery. We lacked the impact of regular, successfully performed major laparoscopic operations to wake up the "coelio-indifferent," to obtain the definitive adhesion of the "coelio-skeptical" and to break apart the *a priori* convictions of the "anti-laparoscopy-by-principle" people. This indeed happened on April 24, 1989, when one of our group presented the laparoscopic cholecystectomy [5] technique at the annual congress of SAGES, in Louisville, Kentucky, in the U.S. In front of an international audience, it was the ideal resonance box for launching the "big-bang" necessary to sweep away all doubts regarding the introduction of laparoscopic surgery to the everyday practice of surgeons all over the world. Laparoscopic cholecystectomy has already been recorded in the history of surgery as being the emblematic operation that opened the gates of minimally invasive surgery.

Chapter 2 of this book, authored by Dr. José Schiappa, relates, as mentioned, to laparoscopic cholecystectomy. This is hardly a surprise for me, since he understood, as did Dr. Cavit Avci, the "big-bang" from Louisville, and both joined EAES where they became representatives of their countries – countries at the most distant extremities of southern Europe, i.e., the western Portugal and eastern Turkey; this is very meaningful. They immediately became our friends and colleagues, taking a very active part in the whole establishment and development of what became EAES, a member of IFSES [6], always bringing improvements in endo-laparoscopic surgery to the rest of the world. Both knew Philippe Mouret very well and had the greatest respect for him, as we all did; this respect definitely deserves an important place in the foreword of their book.

Philippe Mouret is the developer of the technique known as "laparoscopic cholecystectomy," the technique now used by thousands of surgeons all over the world. He successfully completed this operation in his first attempt, in March, 1987, and operated successfully on more than 3,000 patients until his death in 2008. Of course, with the passing of time, and dozens of technical modifications and new instruments – some of them from Philippe Mouret himself – the quality and safety of this operation have improved, but his strategical approach and his original sequence and movements remain the same.

Today, laparoscopic cholecystectomy, which began the "breakthrough" in the spirit of surgeons favoring the use of endoscopes in their everyday practice, is still a strong label of creativity. It is often a research model for testing the validity and interest of a new instrument and of a new operative technique. It was the first laparoscopic procedure designated as the "gold standard" for the treatment of gallbladder lithiasis by the NIH [7] in Bethesda, Maryland, in September 1992. At the beginning of the twenty-first century we were still surprised, together with Philippe

Mouret, to find so many papers in the medical literature relating to complications from this surgery, already so standardized. With all the evidence, José Schiappa shows us that there is always progress to be made in this area. In his chapter, he describes the benefits that modern imaging has brought for detecting anatomical variations in the biliary tree, important preoperative knowledge necessary for preventing peroperative lesions. He shows in detail new strategies and the "tips and tricks" of the operating procedures related both to prevention and to repair.

Chapter 3 is devoted to the treatment of gastro-esophageal reflux, a complex pathology of which some components raise questions that are always interesting and timely. Let us remember that in chronological historical order, during the last decade of the twentieth century, some of the fundoplication procedures were the second to obtain their homologations immediately after laparoscopic cholecystectomy. However, new minimally invasive techniques are arising, using the endolumenal approach. Dr. Cavit Avci approaches these difficult and still-pending problems in a thorough way, focusing his view on the study of complications.

Chapters 4, 5, 6, and 7. In addition to the analysis above, it is necessary to point out that each author has fully respected the pre-established writing guidelines agreement as per the title of the book about complications; as such, it would be repetitive to mention the contents chapter by chapter. All are as informative as the first three chapters. Kudos to the authors, all internationally known and recognized experts in their fields. It is necessary, however, to emphasize the precision and pertinence of the choice of bibliographic references and of the schematic illustrations throughout the entire book. In addition, illustrating the texts with video clips manages to show the updating of this book's pedagogic quality, since studying surgery is at first understanding the correct mandatory maneuvers to be done to perfection, through animated images in order to reproduce them properly at the time of actual surgery.

*In conclusion*: This book gives a good picture of what has become the "state of the art" of seven major procedures of laparoscopic surgery – nowadays classified as "*conventional*." The book will find its place in university libraries, training and educational centers for endoscopic surgery, as well as in the personal libraries of residents in abdominal surgery. It will also interest surgeons already involved in daily practice and concerned with their obligations of continuing education. With the up-to-date information that it contains, this book also consolidates the platform for launching innovative research programs devoted to building the future of surgery as it is done in institutes for advanced education and research in minimally invasive surgery [8, 9].

We wish the book great success.

Doctor Jacques Périssat MD, PHD, FACS
Emeritus Professor of Digestive Surgery
University Victor Segalen, Bordeaux France
Member of the National Academy of Surgery, Paris
Honorary Member of the American Surgical Association

# Bibliographic References

1.  Le Journal de coelio-chirurgie founded in 1992, Edmond Estour chief Editor www.coelio-sur-gery.com
2.  Bruhat MA (1994) Coeliochirurgie: Véritable avancée chirurgicale ou simple tentation du pos-sible. Bull Acad Natl Med 178:199
3.  *EAES*: European Association for Endoscopic Surgery. Founded in 1990 www.eaes-eur.org
4.  *SAGES*: Society American Gastro-intestinal Endoscopic Surgeons. Founded in 1981 www.sages.org
5.  Périssat J, Collet D, Belliard R (1989) Gallstones: laparoscopic treatment by intracorporeal lithotripsy followed by cholecystectomy or cholecystectomy. A personal technique. Endoscopy 21:373–374
6.  *IFSES*: International Federation Societies Endoscopic Surgeons. Founded in 1992 www.ifses.org
7.  Perissat J (1993) Laparoscopic cholecystectomy: The European Experience. Presented at the NIH consensus conference on gallstones and Laparoscopic cholecystectomy, Bethesda Maryland USA September 14–16, 1992. Am J Surg 165:444–449
8.  European School of Laparoscopic Surgery G-B. Cadière President and Director: www.lap-surgery.com
9.  IRCAD France J. Marescaux President and Director: www.ircad.fr

# Acknowledgements

The editors acknowledge the surgeons who have anonymously provided the video clips shown with complications. Since all surgeries have complications, it is extremely important that the video clips, like those shown in this book, be used for educational purposes. We recognize the importance of exposing complications that have occurred in order to understand what went wrong and what can be done to improve surgical safety.

The editors also acknowledge the work of Ms. Carol Anne W. Guerreiro and Dr. Diamantino Guerreiro, who reviewed all texts written by non-English-speaking authors.

José M. Schiappa thanks Ms. Mafalda Penedo (mafaldapenedo@avenidadesign.pt), the artist who drew the figures presented in this chapter, for her help and involvement. Also, special thanks go to Dr. J. Roque for the photo that he provided.

# Contents

# Table of Contents for Videos

Electronic supplementary material is available in the online version of the related chapter on SpringerLink: http://link.springer.com/

# Introduction

Since the first cases on laparoscopic surgery published and presented to the surgical community at the end of the 1980s there has been an enormous "explosion" of its practice all over the world. Depending upon the progress of surgery in each country, this introduction was either a little faster or slower, but soon every country had someone using the approach; however, together with the introduction of the approach came problems.

Many of the surgeons using the new technique were young and without much surgical experience. This, together with the complete change in the surgical approach, led to many complications that were already quite reduced in "classic," open surgery – namely in cholecystectomy, where the rate of lesions to the biliary tract increased dramatically.

Progressively, laparoscopic surgery began to be used in other areas, even becoming the "gold standard" approach for some of these pathologies. Examples are, besides laparoscopic cholecystectomy, the surgical treatment of GERD, and non-traumatic colorectal and spleen surgery. Also here, the rate of complications showed that a great deal of attention had to be given to the education and training of all surgeons involved. When laparoscopic surgery began, most training was done through short courses; many were Industry-related and were followed by surgeons willing to jump on the "laparoscopy wagon," invited there by the industry. These courses, mostly, were not certified and were not teaching in depth or correctly, all of the necessary details on how to perform laparoscopic surgery safely.

This can explain the need that many people think is absolutely necessary to impose: to re-evaluate all teaching programs in laparoscopic surgery and keep offering duly validated training courses and conference discussions on how to minimize the dangers of specific types of this approach.

The impact of these changes can make the difference between high and low rates of complications and iatrogenic lesions in laparoscopic surgery. It has been shown that no surgeon is immune to the possibility of having iatrogenic lesions develop during at least one such surgery; besides, the so-called "learning curve," considered by many to be the main cause of complications, has proven to be not so. Many complications occur in the "consolidated" phase of a surgery; there are several reasons for this, and the texts in this book address that.

- *The risk goes beyond "first cases"; first 1284 cases (in a single Institution) – 0.58 % / following 1143 cases – 0.50 % (Morgenstren et al., Am Surg, 1995)*
- *Enquiry to 1500 surgeons – about 30 % of BDIs occurred after the first 200 cases (Calvete et al., Surg Endosc 2000)*
- *Surgeon's experience does not minimize the risk; without safety measures and careful acting, every surgeon can be struck by one of these complications.*

Learning curve and incidence of iatrogenic lesions

| |
|---|
| Laparoscopy France (24,300 patients) 0.27 % USA (77,600 patients) 0.6 % |
| Portugal (14,455 patients) 0.25 % |
| Italy (13,718 patients) 0.24 % |
| Metanalises 0.8–1 % |
| Laparotomy Johns Hopkins (H.Pitt) 0.1–0.2 % San Diego (A.R.Moossa) 0.5 % |
| Paul-Brousse (H.Bismuth) 0.2 % |
| Cornell Univ. (L.Blumgart) 0.2 % |
| Port. Soc. Surg. (B.Castelo) 0.55 % |

This explains the purpose of this book: to help, as much as possible, to minimize some of these problems. In the various chapters we try to give some advice on the possible complications of each type of surgery and a few "tips and tricks" on how to avoid them. Each chapter is complemented by video clips showing examples of complications of surgical approaches to the pathology the author addresses. We suggest that readers look carefully at the video clips and try to identify the mistakes being made. It is also possible to try to find out, beforehand, what is going to happen as the video clip runs and what can be done to avoid the complication.

These video clips are from real surgeries that were given to us by the surgeons who performed them, during which there were complications; they were given for educational purposes. We thank them for providing the clips, and it goes without saying that that these – anonymous – contributions are crucial for the education of surgeons trying to minimize possible complications. Only the realization that any surgeon can be a protagonist, but for different reasons and, as such, cause a serious complication, will provide us with the capabilities of understanding the absolute need to act in a constant, safe way.

Istanbul, Turkey                                              Cavit Avci
Lisbon, Portugal                                        José M. Schiappa

# Creating the Pneumoperitoneum

Levent Avtan

## 1.1 Starting the Pneumoperitoneum

Pneumoperitoneum is the most commonly used method to obtain exposure of the peritoneal cavity for laparoscopy. Expanding the abdominal cavity by insufflation provides adequate surgical exposure and allows the operative manipulations required in laparoscopic surgery. The most common mode of establishing a pneumoperitoneum is insufflation of carbon dioxide.

Pneumoperitoneum-associated risk factors in laparoscopic surgery may be investigated in two fundamental processes [1]:

- Access and exposure-related risk factors and complications
- Pneumoperitoneum-associated alterations and complications

Despite gasless laparoscopic surgery that has been developed to overcome the potential adverse effects of pneumoperitoneum especially on pregnant (on the foetus) and on geriatric patients, carbon dioxide ($CO_2$) pneumoperitoneum is still the most widely used method [2, 3].

**Electronic supplementary material** The online version of this chapter (doi:10.1007/978-3-319-19623-7_1) contains supplementary material, which is available to authorized users.

L. Avtan, MD
Istanbul School of Medicine, İstanbul University Continuing Medical Education
and Research Centre, Turkish National Association for Endoscopic Laparoscopic Surgery,
Istanbul, Turkey
e-mail: leventavtan@gmail.com

© Springer International Publishing Switzerland 2016
C. Avci, J.M. Schiappa (eds.), *Complications in Laparoscopic Surgery:*
*A Guide to Prevention and Management*, DOI 10.1007/978-3-319-19623-7_1

## 1.1.1  Access to Peritoneal Cavity and Exposure

Generally, carbon dioxide is insufflated at a high rate (up to 15 L/min) to a pressure limit of 12–16 mmHg. However, adjustments are made for age, size and as intraoperative monitoring dictates [4, 5]. As a pressure guideline:

Infant: 4–6 mmHg, insufflation rate less than 1 L/min
Child: 6–8 mmHg, insufflation rate around 1 L/min
Adult: 12–16 mmHg, insufflation rate less than 15 L/min

**A variety of methods of primary peritoneal entry is available:**
Noninsufflated entry method
    Direct trocar and cannula
    Open trocar and cannula
Pre-insufflated entry method with Veress needle
    Conventional closed trocar and cannula
    Shielded trocar and cannula
    Radially expanding trocar and cannula
Visual entry method (with or without pre-insufflation)
    Visual Veress needle
    Visual disposable trocar and cannula
    Visual reusable (EndoTIP) cannula

### 1.1.1.1 The Open Method

Open placement technique was first demonstrated in the United States by Hasson in 1975 and in Germany by Koenig in 1979. It is the safest method of initial port placement. Its use is not limited to initial port placement; any number of ports can be placed using this technique at any location in the abdomen. Some prefer to use this technique in selected cases such as slender, muscular patients, those with prior abdominal procedures or paediatric patients.

The initial port is usually placed at the umbilicus, as this is the thinnest part of the abdominal wall even in muscular or obese patients. If the patient has had a previous midline incision, the second most commonly accepted area to place the initial port is the left upper quadrant. However, placement off the midline in an obese individual can be dauntingly difficult or require an excessively large incision. Placing the incision within the umbilicus yields the most cosmetic scar. By placing the endoscope into the cannula but not through it, proper placement can again be confirmed prior to insufflation. Hasson technique is particularly helpful in patients who have had multiple previous abdominal operations, in whom the risk of adhesions is increased. In some cases, adhesions may be so extensive as to require conversion to laparotomy.

### 1.1.1.2 The Veress Needle

Prior to blind placement of the Veress needle or trocars into the peritoneal cavity, the bladder and stomach are emptied, and the aorta palpated to decrease the chance of injury. The snap mechanism of the Veress needle is checked. A skin incision large enough to fit the ensuing trocar is made, and the subcutaneous tissues are bluntly dissected down to the anterior fascia. Generally, the spring mechanism will snap three times as the Veress needle penetrates the fascial layers and the peritoneum, while all resistance disappears once the peritoneal cavity is entered. The Veress needle should be freely mobile through 360°.

*Testing* A number of tests have been devised to confirm placement in the peritoneal cavity. Injected saline flows freely and aspiration is freely accomplished returning neither blood nor enteric contents. The "slurp" test – A drop of saline placed in the closed Veress needle should flow freely once the needle is opened, especially if the abdominal wall is lifted.

The insufflation tubing may then be attached and started on low flow. Patient's pressure reading should be low with free flow of gas and symmetric insufflation of the abdominal cavity. This serves as further confirmation of proper placement. A "visual Veress needle" is also on the market that further confirms proper placement using a thin endoscope that fits through the needle.

### 1.1.1.3 Trocar Placement Without Prior Pneumoperitoneum (Sharp/Bladeless)

Some surgeons advocate simple blind trocar placement with manual counter traction on the abdominal wall without prior pneumoperitoneum. However, it is better to use bladeless trocar under visual guidance of a laparoscope.

Regardless of the mode, once access is obtained, the first step is to inspect the peritoneal cavity to rule out iatrogenic injury.

## 1.2 Access and Exposure-Related Risk Factors

### 1.2.1 Improper Placement of the Veress Needle

**Prevention** If one is not initially convinced of proper placement, due to failing one or more of the above-mentioned tests, one or two additional attempts at placement may be made. Then open placement technique should be undertaken.

### 1.2.2 Sudden Uncontrolled Entry into the Peritoneal Cavity

**Prevention** Apply traction on the towel clips or directly retract the abdominal wall with one hand. Place the needle perpendicularly through the anterior abdominal wall under gentle controlled pressure, with the dominant hand resting on the abdominal wall, holding the needle not at the handle, but slightly closer to the tip.

### 1.2.3    High-Pressure Reading

If one is certain of proper placement but the pressure reading is too high, other causes for this include water in the tubing, closed valves, kinking of the tubing or inadequate relaxation of the patient.

Once the abdominal cavity is adequately insufflated, remove the needle, and place a sharp or dilating trocar with counter traction on the towel clips or by directly grasping and lifting the abdominal wall. After introducing the trocar, remove its inside part, keeping the outside cannula on place. Confirm the correct placement by the endoscope, and the insufflation tubing can be reconnected.

### 1.2.4    Poor Visualisation

**Cause** Decreased light due to slightly bloodier nature of potential spaces or dirty scope.

**Management** Increase intensity or gain of light; irrigate and suction the area. Frequently clean the lens with anti-fog solution and warm water as there are no proper peritoneal surfaces on which to wipe the scope.

### 1.2.5    Risks-Related Port Location

The most important factors in placing the ports are to space them in such a way that they do not interfere with each other and to trying to keep instruments in line with the camera. One rule of thumb is that the distance between the cannula and the operative site should be approximately half the length of the instrument. Ports are generally placed in a loosely configured semicircle around the operative site, although personal experience and specific patient factors may require a different number and configuration than routinely recommended. In the midline, the falciform ligament can get in the way superiorly, and the bladder can be injured inferiorly. More laterally, one risks injuring the epigastric vessels. Placing a port in the flanks risks damage to the colon. Excessive pressure at any site risks damage to all underlying organs and vessels.

**Prevention** Transilluminate abdominal wall prior to trocar placement. The anatomy of the abdominal wall as well as underlying organs must be considered.

### 1.2.6    Uncontrolled Entry

**Prevention** The skin incision should be one to two millimetres larger than the trocar. The trocar is generally placed with a twisting motion, applying pressure with the wrist, not the shoulder. The middle or index finger is extended along the trocar to prevent uncontrolled entry. The trocar is angled slightly towards the operative field, but not to a degree as for the trocar to slide along the outside of the peritoneum. Previously the "Z" placement technique was widely used to decrease leakage of pneumoperitoneum. Although this is less of a problem with newer trocars and grips, this technique may be useful in certain patients undergoing lengthy procedures.

### 1.2.7 Removal of Cannulas

Cannulas must be removed under direct visualisation, as a vessel may be tamponed with haemorrhage manifesting only after removal (Video 1.1). The operative field should be inspected under decreased pressure since bleeding may be tamponed by the pneumoperitoneum pressure and only become manifest once this is released.

Video 1.1: Trocar site bleeding 90 s

## 1.3 Access and Exposure-Related Complications

Complications of the Veress needle or blind placement techniques include vascular, gastrointestinal, urological and gynaecological trauma, as well as damage to solid organs. Although less frequent, these complications are not eliminated by using the open technique. If initial attempts to prevent or treat complications are unsuccessful, immediate cessation of the operation or conversion to laparotomy should be performed.

### 1.3.1 Preperitoneal Insufflation

**Cause** Placement of the Veress needle at too great an angle or trocar sliding out into the preperitoneal space (Video 1.2).

**Prevention** Place Veress needle perpendicularly and pass all tests, and place trocars securely and check placement prior to insufflation.

**Management** Replace Veress needle or trocar, secure trocar with an additional fascial suture, convert to open procedure and allow time for resolution.

Video 1.2: Preperitoneal insufflation 54 s

### 1.3.2 Piercing the Greater Omentum with the Veress Needle

This can cause bleeding or produce interstitial emphysema of the greater omentum, pushing it against the anterior abdominal wall with insufflation.

**Prevention** Make sure the abdominal wall is lifted during insertion of the Veress needle. Advance the tip less than one cm after the last audible snap of the Veress needle, rotate the needle and perform the safety tests.

**Management** This complication is often recognised only after inserting the endoscope. Once recognised, withdraw the trocar to the level of the peritoneum then gently tap the abdominal wall from the outside to return the omentum to its original position. Control of omental bleeding can usually be performed laparoscopically.

### 1.3.3  Puncture of a Hollow Organ with the Veress Needle

The "slurp" and rotation tests are generally not successful in this situation.

**Prevention** Do not insert the Veress needle near laparotomy scars. Pay strict attention to all positioning tests.

**Management** If you can bring the trocar back into the peritoneal cavity, an attempt to remove the carbon dioxide by aspiration through a fine needle may be made with laparoscopic repair of the injury. If unsuccessful, conversion to laparotomy is indicated.

## 1.4     Complications of Potential Space Exposure

Such areas include "the preperitoneal space" for hernia repair and urologic procedures; "the retroperitoneal space" for neurologic, vascular, orthopaedic or urologic procedures; and "the subfascial plane" in the leg for vascular procedures where no space actually exists. A variety of balloon dissectors is available. The principles of the procedure for entering the preperitoneal space may generally be applied to any area.

### 1.4.1  Haemorrhage

**Prevention** Completely retract all strands of muscle laterally and cauterise any visible vessels.

### 1.4.2  Uneven Inflation

If the balloon inflates unevenly, or more dissection is needed unilaterally, manual pressure on the contralateral abdominal wall with further inflation of the balloon is sometimes of benefit.

### 1.4.3 Violation of the Peritoneal Cavity

**Prevention** Direct the balloon dissector against the peritoneum when advancing it.

**Management** Close the defect by suturing or clipping. Attempt placement on contralateral side or avoid defect and continue with procedures.

## 1.5 Complications of Trocar Placement

The visually controlled insertion of working ports for the operative instruments and retractors are important. More than 10 % of laparoscopic complications are associated with trocar insertion [6].

### 1.5.1 Abdominal Wall Haemorrhage

**Cause** Laceration of abdominal wall vessel. The source of bleeding is usually the inferior epigastric artery or one of its branches.

**Prevention** Transilluminate abdominal wall prior to trocar placement. Using the bladeless trocars minimises the risk by dilating the tissue while entering. Abdominal wall haemorrhage may be controlled with a variety of technique, including application of direct pressure with operating port, open or laparoscopic suture ligation, or apply pressure with a Foley catheter inserted into the peritoneal cavity.

**Management** The trocar should be removed and the vessel cauterised externally or internally or ligated through an enlarged incision. The trocar is then replaced. Otherwise, the trocar may be removed with closure of the fascia and placement of the trocar elsewhere. Alternatively, a Foley balloon can be placed, inflated and retracted to tampon the bleeding. This method is time consuming, and if unsuccessful, one of the previously mentioned options must be undertaken. To understand the bleeding comes through which side, cantilever the trocar into each quadrant to find a position that causes the bleeding to stop. When the proper quadrant is found, pressure from the portion of the sheath within the abdomen tampons the bleeding vessel, thus stopping the bleeding. Then place a suture in such a manner that it traverses the entire border of the designated quadrant. Specialised devices have been made that facilitate placement of a suture but are not always readily available. The needle should enter the abdomen on one side of the trocar and exit on the other side, thereby encircling the full thickness of the abdominal wall. This suture can be passed percutaneously either using a large curved # 1 absorbable suture as monitored endoscopically or using a straight Keith needle passed into the abdomen and then back out using laparoscopic grasping forceps. The suture, which encircles the abdominal wall, is tied over a gauze bolster to tampon the bleeding site.

## 1.5.2 Major Vascular Injury

**Cause** Excessive pressure without adequate visualisation. Major vascular injury can occur when the sharp tip of the Veress needle or the trocar nicks or lacerates a mesenteric or retroperitoneal vessel. It is rare when the open (Hasson cannula) technique is used.

**Prevention** Controlled trocar placement under direct visualisation without undue pressure.

**Management** If aspiration of the Veress needle reveals bloody fluids, remove the needle and puncture again the abdomen. Once access to the abdominal cavity has been achieved successfully, perform a full examination of the retroperitoneum to look for an expanding retroperitoneal haematoma. If there is a central or expanding retroperitoneal haematoma, laparotomy with retroperitoneal exploration is mandatory to access for and repair major vascular injury. Haematomas of the mesentery and those located laterally in the retroperitoneum are generally innocuous and may be just controlled by observation. If during closed insertion of the initial trocar there is a rush of blood through the trocar with associated hypotension, leave the trocar in place (to provide some tamponing of the haemorrhage and to assist in identifying the tract) and immediately perform laparotomy to repair what is likely to be an injury to the aorta, vena cava or iliac vessels. Minimal: pressure and thrombogens. Moderate or continued: if expertise is available, and the bleeding site clearly seen, then a maximum of two attempts may be made to control the bleeding by applying clips, ligatures or suturing. Heavy, continued or expertise not available: immediate conversion to laparotomy.

## 1.5.3 Bowel Injury

**Prevention** Careful observation of the steps enumerated will minimise the chance of visceral injury. However, placement of the Veress needle is a blind manoeuvre,

| Factors responsible for large vessel injury | Inexperienced or unskilled surgeon |
|---|---|
| | Failure to sharpen the trocar |
| | Failure to elevate or stabilise the abdominal wall |
| | Perpendicular insertion of the needle or trocar |
| | Lateral deviation of the needle or trocar |
| | Inadequate pneumoperitoneum |
| | Forceful thrust |
| | Failure to note anatomical landmarks |
| | Inadequate incision size |

and even with extreme care, puncture of a hollow viscus is still possible. Once the peritoneal cavity has been entered, the trocar can be angled anteriorly to avoid potential danger to underlying organs.

**Management** If aspiration of the Veress needle returns yellowish or cloudy fluid, the needle is likely in the lumen of the bowel. Due to small calibre of the needle itself, this is usually a harmless situation. Simply remove the needle and puncture again the abdominal wall. After successful insertion of the laparoscope, examine the abdominal viscera closely for significant injury. If, however, the laparoscopic trocar itself lacerates the bowel, the injured area can sometimes be withdrawn through the incision and repaired extracorporeally or repaired intracorporeally depending on the experience of the surgeon. There are four possible courses of action: formal open laparotomy and bowel repair or resection; mini-laparotomy, using an incision just large enough to exteriorise the injured bowel segment for repair or resection and reanastomosis; laparoscopic resection of injured bowel and reanastomosis; and laparoscopic suture repair of the bowel injury. If possible, leave the trocar in place to assist in identifying the precise site of injury [7].

### 1.5.4 Bladder Injury

**Prevention** Controlled trocar placement under direct visualisation, empty the bladder prior to procedure.

**Management** Damage to any organ is treated in a fashion similar to that for blood vessel injury. Two attempts if the expertise is available, otherwise, open. Drain the area and administer antibiotics as indicated.

### 1.6 Trauma Related with the Type of Port

The ports should be chosen with the specific procedure in mind, taking into account the surgeon's preference, cost and what exact instrumentation will be needed.

There are many different trocar tips available, each with its own benefits and limitations. Pyramidal tips are reputed to cause more damage than conical tips; however, conical tips require excessive force to introduce. The knife blade tip theoretically causes less abdominal wall trauma; however, it cannot be introduced using the usual twisting method. Reusable trocars may become dull over time (Video 1.3).

Video 1.3: Injury risk related with the type of port 60 s

Many feel that shielded trocars are safer; however, they do not tend to be as easily introduced, leading to a greater amount of pressure being applied. The shield is supposed to pop out and lock around the blade once the trocar has entered the abdomen. However, if the skin incision is too small, the shield may be held back. Newer shielded trocars with a blade that retracts into the shield should eliminate this problem. Some newer cannulas minimise dangers associated with trocars. One is a disposable expandable sleeve, which is introduced using the Veress needle and then dilated to the necessary size using a blunt introducer. The other is a reusable threaded cannula, which is introduced through a small incision in the anterior fascia. Using rotational force, under direct vision, it bluntly dissects its way into abdomen. Another one is a disposable cannula with a bladeless trocar that is introduced under laparoscopic view by dilating the tissues. Both are reported to decrease trauma to the abdominal wall structures, as well as leaving smaller defects to close. No matter which product is used, careful controlled entry is the key.

## 1.7 Pneumoperitoneum-Associated Complications

### 1.7.1 Cardiopulmonary Trouble

**Prevention**  Keep the insufflation pressure and time to a minimum, proper patient selection.

**Management**  Evacuate the pneumoperitoneum. Cease the procedure if not too far advanced, convert to laparotomy if necessary, use adequate fluid resuscitation.

### 1.7.2 Gas Embolisation

**Prevention**  Use the lowest insufflation pressure compatible with adequate visualisation, reduce operating time, release pneumoperitoneum when not actively working.

**Management**  Evacuate pneumoperitoneum, left lateral decubitus position, 100 % oxygen, aspiration through central venous catheter, if catheter was previously placed [8].

### 1.7.3 Localised Collection of Carbon Dioxide

Manually deflate or aspirate prior to end of procedure.

### 1.7.4 Deep Vein Thrombosis

**Prevention**  Use antithrombotic pneumatic sleeves on lower extremities, low-dose heparin prophylaxis, keep pneumoperitoneum insufflation pressure and duration to a minimum.

## 1.7.5 Postoperative Shoulder or Subphrenic Pain

**Cause** Alterations in the physiological environment of the peritoneal cavity may explain postoperative shoulder pain. Potential causes are the temperature of the gas used for the pneumoperitoneum as it leaves the storage cylinder (usually 20 °C), irritation of the diaphragm due to muscular distension as well as chemical reactions by gas on the peritoneum. Carbon dioxide is irritating to the peritoneum.

**Prevention** Warming the gas to body temperature as it is insufflated and taking care to completely evacuate the peritoneal cavity may decrease pain. Other gases such as nitrous oxide have anaesthetic properties on the peritoneum; however, potential danger of combustion limits their widespread use.

Patients should be warned preoperatively that they may have shoulder pain (around 25 % of all patients) and that this will subside spontaneously within 2–3 days without analgesic treatment.

## 1.8    Pneumoperitoneum-Associated Physiologic Alterations

Cardiovascular/haemodynamic and pulmonary changes associated with the pneumoperitoneum represent a complex balance between the factors mentioned above. Carbon dioxide insufflation may also affect acid-base balance and may lead to further deterioration of existing intraperitoneal sepsis or inflammation.

**Factors Influencing Haemodynamic and Pulmonary Changes During laparoscopic Surgery**

- Mechanical effects of increased intra-abdominal pressure
- Systemic effects of absorbed gas
- Control of hypercarbia through augmentation of minute ventilation
- Intravascular volume status
- Body positioning (Trendelenburg and reverse-Trendelenburg positions)
- Anaesthetic technique
- Degree of surgical or pain stimulus
- Cardiovascular comorbidity

## 1.9    Mechanical Effects of Increased Intra-abdominal Pressure

Insufflation of the abdominal cavity and elevation of intra-abdominal pressure have three predominant mechanical effects on cardiovascular functions:

- Increased afterload
- Increased venous resistance
- Increased mean systemic pressure

Isolated elevation of intra-abdominal pressure produces compression of the splanchnic circulation, resulting in increased afterload and depression of cardiac function.

The increased abdominal pressure has an effect similar to positive end-expiratory pressure (PEEP) on haemodynamic variables. Thus, in animal studies, a decrease in cardiac output with concomitant increase of the central venous pressure and the peripheral systemic vascular resistance was observed after implementation of pneumoperitoneum [9]. Some other studies did not report on significant changes in cardiac output, while mean arterial pressure, systemic vascular resistance and central venous pressure were elevated [10].

In high-risk cardiac patients, the effect of $CO_2$ pneumoperitoneum is more pronounced as compared to healthy individuals [11]. In addition, another study showed a decrease in heart rate and cardiac output without the compensatory mechanism of an elevated systemic venous resistance. The authors suggested that mixed venous oxygen saturation is the most sensitive parameter in monitoring cardiovascular function [12].

Pressure-related effects of pneumoperitoneum include decreased blood flow through the inferior vena cava. This in turn leads to reduced filling volume and pressure in the right and left atrium with consequent decrease in preload. According to the Frank-Starling law, this effect can be compensated up to a point after which the cardiac output falls. Increases in central venous pressure due to higher intrathoracic pressure during mechanical ventilation and additional pneumoperitoneum falsely suggest sufficient volume status. Therefore, a decrease in cardiac output is the sequel of decreased preload, which is compensated by an increase in afterload from a rise in systemic venous resistance. The net effect is a stable or slightly decreased cardiac output and mean arterial pressure under normal conditions, i.e. adequate cardiac reserve and sufficient volume status. There is evidence that increasing intra-abdominal pressure decreases splanchnic blood flow, which adversely affects mucosal microcirculation.

Another study showed significant correlation between increasing intra-abdominal pressure and decreasing gastric mucosal pH measured by tonometry during $CO_2$ pneumoperitoneum in a porcine model [13]. These results were interpreted as significant end-organ impairment, while at the same time significant differences in macrocirculatory parameters such as heart rate, cardiac output, pulmonary capillary wedge pressure and central venous pressure were not observed.

## 1.10 Direct Systemic Effects of Absorbed CO₂

Transperitoneal absorption of $CO_2$ is the main cause of hypercapnia when a $CO_2$ pneumoperitoneum is established [14]. Hypercapnia has several effects on the cardiovascular system (Table 1.1).

Mild hypercapnia may lead to an increase in systemic venous resistance, thus increasing cardiac output and mean arterial pressure, while extensive hypercapnia causes depression of cardiac function [15]. After establishing a $CO_2$ pneumoperitoneum,

**Table 1.1** $CO_2$ pneumoperitoneum-related effects on cardiovascular function

**Absorption of CO₂ (Hypercapnia)**

- Dissolved $CO_2$ Acidosis (Arrhythmias)

  Mild Acidemia (Sympathetic stimulation); Increased MAP, HR, SVR
  Severe Acidemia (Negative inotropic effect); depressed left ventricular function

**Pressure of Gas**

- Mechanical effect of increased IP (Compression of venous structures) ⎤ Decreased Preload
- Position of patient (Trendelenburg and Reverse Trendelenburg) ⎦ (Venous Return)

*MAP* mean arterial pressure, *HR* heart rate, *SVR* systemic vascular resistant, *IP* intraperitoneal pressure

the systemic $CO_2$ concentration rises due to the partial pressure difference between intraperitoneal $CO_2$ and capillary blood pressure, leading to diffusion of $CO_2$ into the blood. The resulting hypercapnia augments respiratory frequency and tidal volume in order to excrete the additional $CO_2$. These compensatory mechanisms warrant an intact buffering system. In sick patients, however, additional $CO_2$ might overwhelm this system and augment preexisting acidosis (e.g. in septic patients). Thus, a $CO_2$ pneumoperitoneum in severe abdominal sepsis may be detrimental and should, therefore, be avoided [16]. This aspect may have significant implications considering reports on laparoscopic repair of hollow viscus perforations [17]. There are somewhat contradictory reports on changes in $pO_2$ during laparoscopy. Effects of the pneumoperitoneum vary from decrease to no change to an increase in $pO_2$. These discrepancies may be explained by the Trendelenburg position of the patient and different modes of ventilation between groups of patients. While patients who are breathing spontaneously show a lower $pO_2$, patients on the respirator have an elevated $pO_2$ probably due to a higher $FiO_2$. The changes in pulmonary function occurring during a $CO_2$ pneumoperitoneum are summarised in Table 1.2 [18].

In comparison to an open operation, postoperative pulmonary function seems to be better after laparoscopy. Frazee and co-workers reported a better pulmonary function postoperatively in patients undergoing laparoscopic cholecystectomy as compared to patients undergoing open surgery [19].

## 1.11 Pneumoperitoneum and Abdominal Sepsis

Following the rapid acceptance of elective laparoscopic cholecystectomy, additional applications for minimal invasive surgery have been sought. Amongst these, laparoscopic closure of peptic ulcer perforation has been added to our operative armamentarium [17]. However, in conditions related to peritonitis, some experimental evidence has drawn attention to a theoretical risk concerning the $CO_2$ pneumoperitoneum [20, 21].

Laparoscopic surgical techniques require distension and elevation of the abdominal wall from the viscera to allow visualisation and manipulation. In the clinical

**Table 1.2** $CO_2$ pneumoperitoneum-related changes in pulmonary function

| Pulmonary function | Change |
|---|---|
| Peak inspiratory pressure (PIP) | Up |
| Pulmonary compliance (dV/dT) | Down |
| Vital capacity (VC) | Down |
| Functional residual capacity (FRC) | Down |
| Intrathoracic pressure (ITP) | Up |

**Table 1.3** Laparoscopy-related peritoneal alterations

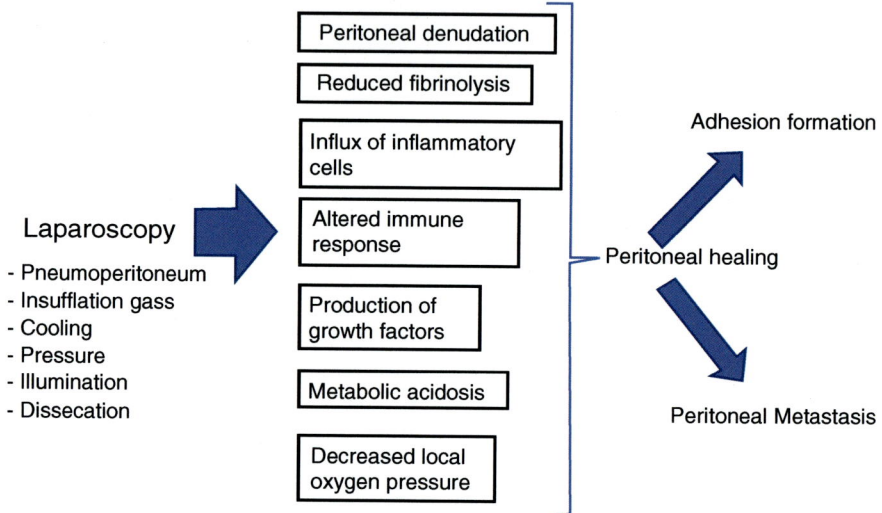

situation, this is generally realised by intraperitoneal gas insufflation and maintenance of a continuous positive intra-abdominal pressure of approximately 8–12 mmHg. As observed in an experimental study, distension of the abdominal wall imposed by a pneumoperitoneum results in temporary stretching of the parietal mesothelial cells with concomitant flat bending of microvilli. Normal conformation of the mesothelium returns within 2 h after release of the pneumoperitoneum [16]. Increased intra-abdominal pressure due to the use of carbon dioxide insufflation apparently leads to the same ultrastructural changes observed after saline injection [22]. Thus, it may be concluded that it is the increased intra-abdominal pressure rather than a specific agent or gas that causes the described changes (Table 1.3).

The parietal peritoneum physiologically functions as a barrier with controlled pathways to remove fluids, particles and cells from the peritoneal cavity. Abdominal secretions are drained by large terminal lymphatics that are located beneath the mesothelium of the peritoneal surface of the diaphragm. The absorbed fluid is then transported to the venous system by the thoracic duct. Increased intra-abdominal pressure has been shown to increase the resorption rate of intraperitoneal secretions [22, 23].

Furthermore, inflammatory stimuli are known to cause marked changes of the ultrastructural integrity of the mesothelial cell layer. Shrinking of mesothelial cells leads to disintegration and opening of the latticed intercellular network [22].

The combination of increased intra-abdominal pressure due to the $CO_2$ pneumoperitoneum and of a gastric perforation with secondary inflammation results in premature deterioration of mesothelial integrity. The process of destruction includes numerical reduction as well as shrinking and coarsening of otherwise abundantly present microvilli. Furthermore, mesothelial cellular continuity is interrupted allowing the formation of stomata to the submesothelial cell layer. These changes to the ultrastructural anatomy of the mesothelial cell layer impair the barrier function of the parietal peritoneum giving way to uncontrolled resorption of abdominal secretions, which may induce bacteraemia, endotoxaemia and ultimately septic shock [16].

Based on these observations, experimental evidence demonstrating an aggravation of peritonitis and sepsis in conditions related to severe, long-lasting peritonitis is substantiated [20]. In contrast, another experimental setting in which the interval between bacterial inoculation and onset of pneumoperitoneum lasted only 60 min did not reveal any adverse effects [21].

Regarding both the available experimental and clinical evidence, a considerable risk for a pneumoperitoneum to aggravate peritonitis and to generate septic complications may be anticipated in conditions related to severe abdominal sepsis [24, 25]. Critical appraisal of laparoscopic surgery is warranted in conditions associated with severe, long-standing peritonitis.

## References

1. Lam A, Khong SY, Bignardi T (2010) Principles and strategies for dealing with complications in laparoscopy. Curr Opin Obstet Gynecol 22:315–319
2. Sesti F, Pietropolli A, Sesti FF, Piccione E (2013) Gasless laparoscopic surgery during pregnancy: evaluation of its role and usefulness. Eur J Obstet Gynecol Reprod Biol 170:8–12
3. Li SH, Deng J, Huang FT, Gan XW, Cao YG (2014) Impact of gasless laparoscopy on circulation, respiration, stress response, other complications in gynecological geriatrics. Int J Clin Exp Med 15:2877–2882
4. Cheng Y, Lu J, Xiong X, Wu S, Lin Y, Wu T, Cheng N. Gases for establishing pneumoperitoneum during laparoscopic abdominal surgery. Cochrane Database Syst Rev 2013;31: 1-CD009569
5. Gurusamy KS, Vaughan J, Davidson BR. Low pressure versus standard pressure pneumoperitoneum in laparoscopic cholecystectomy. Cochrane Database Syst Rev 2014;18:3-CD006930
6. Soper NJ, Scott-Corner CEH (eds) (2012) Basic laparoscopy and endoscopy. The SAGES Manual, 3rd edn. Springer, New York
7. Ulker K, Anuk T, Bozkurt M, Karasu Y (2014) Large bowel injuries during gynecological laparoscopy. World J Clin Cases 16:846–851
8. Otsuka Y, Katagiri T, Ishii J, Maeda T, Kubota Y, Tamura A, Tsuchiya M, Kaneko H (2013) Gas embolism in laparoscopic hepatectomy: what is the optimal pneumoperitoneal pressure for laparoscopic major hepatectomy? J Hepatobiliary Pancreat Sci 20:137–140
9. Kashtan J, Green JF, Parsons EQ, Holcroft JW (1981) Hemodynamic effects of increased abdominal pressure. J Surg Res 30:249–255
10. Motew M, Ivankovich AD, Bieniarz J, Albrecht RF, Zahed B, Sommegna A (1973) Cardiovascular effects, acid–base and blood gas changes during laparoscopy. Am J Obstet Gynecol 115:1002–1012
11. Fox LG, Hein H, Gawey B (1993) Physiologic alterations during laparoscopic cholecystectomy. Anesthesiology 79:A55 (Abstract)

12. Safran D, Sganbti S, Orlando R (1993) Laparoscopy in high risk cardiac patients. Surg Gynecol Obstet 176:548–554
13. Knolmayr TJ, Bowyer MW, Egan JC, Asburn HJ (1998) The effect of pneumoperitoneum on gastric blood flow and traditional hemodynamic measurements. Surg Endosc 12:115–118
14. Ho HS, Gunther RA, Wolfe BM (1992) Intraperitoneal carbon dioxide insufflation and cardiopulmonary functions. Arch Surg 127:928–932
15. Marshall RL, Jebson PJR, Davie IT, Scott DB (1972) Circulatory effects of carbon dioxide insufflation of the peritoneal cavity for laparoscopy. Br J Anaesth 44:680–684
16. Bloechle C, Kluth D, Holstein AF, Emmermann A, Strate T, Zornig C, Izbicki JR (1999) A pneumoperitoneum perpetuates severe damage of the ultrastructural integrity of parietal peritoneum in gastric perforation and induced peritonitis in rats. Surg Endosc 13:683–688
17. Mouret P, Francois Y, Vignal J, Barth X, Lombard-Platet R (1990) Laparoscopic treatment of perforated peptic ulcer. Br J Surg 77:1006
18. Safran D, Orlando R (1994) Physiologic effects of pneumoperitoneum. Am Surg 167:281–286
19. Frazee RC, Roberts JW, Okeson GC, Symmonds RE, Synder SK, Hendricks JC, Smith RW (1991) Open versus laparoscopic cholecystectomy: a comparison of postoperative pulmonary function. Ann Surg 213:651–653
20. Evasovich MR, Clark TC, Horattas MC, Holda S, Treen L (1996) Does pneumoperitoneum during laparoscopy increase bacterial translocation? Surg Endosc 10:1176–1179
21. Gurtner GC, Robertson CS, Chung SC, Ling TK, lp SM, Li AK (1995) Effect of carbon dioxide pneumoperitoneum on bacteraemia and endotoxaemia in an animal model of peritonitis. Br J Surg 82:844–848
22. Tsilibary EC, Wissig SL (1983) Lymphatic absorption from the peritoneal cavity: regulation of patency of mesothelial stomata. Microvasc Res 25:22–39
23. Leak LV, Rahil K (1978) Permeability of the diaphragmatic mesothelium: the ultra-structural basis for "stomata". Am J Anat 151:557–594
24. Brokelman WJ, Lensvelt M, Borel Rinkes IH, Klinkenbijl JH, Reijnen MM (2011) Peritoneal changes due to laparoscopic surgery. Surg Endosc 25:1–9
25. Sammour T, Mittal A, Loveday BP, Kahokehr A, Phillips AR, Windsor JA, Hill AG (2009) Systematic review of oxidative stress associated with pneumoperitoneum. Br J Surg 96: 836–850

# Complications in Biliary Surgery: Tips and Tricks

**2**

José M. Schiappa

## 2.1 Problem

Lesions of the biliary tract can happen during the performance of different types of surgery, not only biliary surgery itself. Mainly – although other much rarer options can happen – five types of surgery are responsible for these events:

Biliary surgery
Liver surgery
Portal hypertension surgery
Pancreatic surgery
Gastric surgery

In these types of surgery, sometimes dissection can be difficult, and the surgeon may lose the anatomic landmarks, becoming closer to causing lesions by dissecting and cutting tissue in the areas where the main anatomical structures are, because of not being aware of their real position.

Processes with a serious inflammatory reaction, or the ones which involve large tumours or collateral circulation, or, also very frequently, reoperations causing adhesions and distortion of the local anatomy, make the whole surgical work in that field much more prone to lesions.

Going into a more detailed approach, let us start by looking at the most common biliary surgery performed: cholecystectomy. Our text will be directed at this type of surgery. Some studies rate this problem of iatrogenic lesions at a high stake, but these figures depend on the detail the surgical community relies on in finding

**Electronic supplementary material** The online version of this chapter (doi:10.1007/978-3-319-19623-7_2) contains supplementary material, which is available to authorized users.

J.M. Schiappa, MD, FACS, PhD (Hon)
Department of Surgery, Hospital CUF Infante Santo, Lisbon, Portugal
e-mail: jschiappa@net.vodafone.pt

© Springer International Publishing Switzerland 2016
C. Avci, J.M. Schiappa (eds.), *Complications in Laparoscopic Surgery: A Guide to Prevention and Management*, DOI 10.1007/978-3-319-19623-7_2

**Table 2.1**

| Biliary complications | | Non-biliary complications | |
|---|---|---|---|
| Residual stones | 0.3–18 % | Operative wound (infection) | 0.1–7.9 % |
| Biliary fistulae | 0.1–0.4 % | Haemorrhage | 0.2–2.2 % |
| Biliary tract lesions | 0.1–0.8 % | Respiratory problems | 2.0–5.3 % |
| Pancreatitis | 0.5–1.0 % | Deep vein thrombosis | 0.6–1.3 % |
| | | Bowel occlusion | 0.3–0.7 % |
| | | Vascular stroke | 0.8 % |
| | | Pulmonary embolism | 0.3–1.0 % |

complications and how these are graded; a multicentre study, for instance, of 24.800 patients, relates "post-cholecystectomy symptoms" from 12 to 68 %, and, depending on the centres reporting, serious complications were from 3 to 32 %. These figures show immediately that local approach and reporting are extremely variable and can cause confusion.

Nevertheless, reported rates of morbidity and mortality from cholecystectomy are not very different with the passage of years. Several series show this, with morbidity between 3.8 and 4.9 % and mortality from 0 to 1.8 % [1–3]. In these series, it is noted that a remarkable difference exists in the morbidity and mortality results, dependent, for example, on the age of patients; patients below 65 years of age have much lower mortality rates, for instance [3].

Bile duct injuries (BDI) keep having high incidence, despite all interest given and "calls for attention" which are being made so frequently. Very recently, SAGES set up a "task force" with the task of educating USA surgeons trying to obtain lower rates of lesions ("Safe Cholecystectomy Program"). These rates vary between less than 0.2 and 0.8 % and even more in "normal" cholecystectomies. But, if surgery was performed because of acute cholecystitis, these values are higher.

Even more so, in the difficult cases, leading to "conversion to open". These, interestingly, show very high rates of lesions despite this conversion, which would, in theory, give better "view" to the operating field.

Within cholecystectomy, still the types of complications vary between biliary and non-biliary. Another multicentre study, covering 34.500 patients, showed the following complications and rates, post-cholecystectomy (Table 2.1):

On the whole, a little less than the previous mentioned ones, it is necessary to consider that some patients have more than one complication.

Non-biliary complications are the usual ones, known in general, and possible in any case of abdominal surgery; we are not going to talk about it in this chapter, concentrating our comments on the biliary ones and, amongst these, in the iatrogenic lesions to the biliary tract. These can be detected immediately, during surgery, in the early postoperative period or late, sometimes even months after surgery. What is also important is that about 2/3 of these lesions are not detected during surgery.

Nevertheless, we have to mention that some haemorrhage can be avoided by paying special attention to local factors: for instance, patients with coagulation disturbances or with portal hypertension may have to be dealt with by different solutions

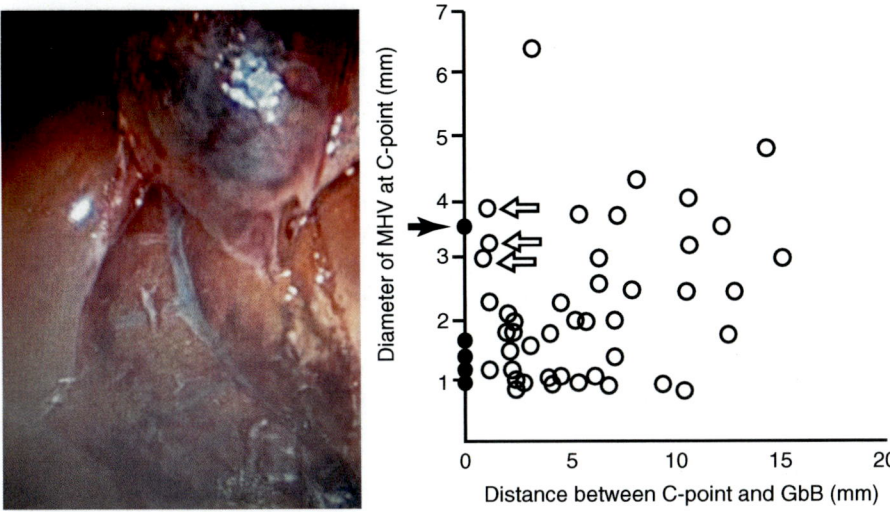

**Fig. 2.1** Vein at gallbladder's bed and its frequency of depth [4] (Photo – courtesy of Dr. Jaime Roque)

like a partial Torek's cholecystectomy. In addition, the draining vein running within liver parenchyma, sometimes rather superficial, in the gallbladder bed, shall be avoided by taking all necessary steps not to go deep during the lifting of the gallbladder from its liver bed [4] (Fig. 2.1). If bleeding comes from this vein, control may be hazardous. The gallbladder shall be dissected from its bed by "lifting" it and by simple separation, without being necessary to do any sharp cutting in general. In cases of acute cholecystitis or of strong adhesions after several inflammatory episodes, this may be necessary, but it is then when all surgeons shall be over attentive and when all cautious movements shall be put into practice.

Obviously, it is supposed that elective patients have a complete workout, where alterations like abnormal blood clotting will be detected and proper measures taken.

Within the biliary complications, the contents of this chapter will focus mainly in the iatrogenic lesions.

## 2.2 Causes ("Why" It May Happen)

If we look at the possible causes of complications, we have several variables to consider. These depend on the patient's general condition and comorbidities, on the type and seriousness of the disease, on the training and expertise of the surgeon, on the quality and existence of all pieces of equipment necessary and on the hospital environment.

Another frequently mentioned variable, in what concerns laparoscopic surgery, is the so-called learning curve. But, although this "learning curve" can be responsible for many things and has to be eliminated or minimised as much as possible, it has no defined causal relation to BDI; the "learning curve" for laparoscopic chole-cystectomy goes well beyond 50 cases, and, although operating time keeps lowering until 200 cases, improvement in the cognitive skills to deal with difficult cases continues [5].

It has also been shown that the risk goes beyond "first cases", as demonstrated in the following series from the same institution: first 1284 cases (0.58 % BDI) and next 1143 cases (0.50 % BDI) [6]. An enquiry into 1500 surgeons reports that about 30 % of BDI occur after the first 200 cases [7]. We can only conclude that surgeon's experience does not minimise the risk.

This persistence of high rates of BDI after the initial training curve shows that there is a difference in these; it is considered that there is a difference between "experienced" surgeons and "experts". "Experts" are surgeons with "consistently better outcomes" (namely, BDI rates, consistent and very low or close to zero).

Some local factors have shown to be responsible for a higher incidence of complications: local inflammation is a well-known one, even conditioning the timing of surgery for acute cholecystitis; fibrosis, reoperations with "changed" anatomy or urgent surgery are other causes. Also, local adhesions or bowel distension can be a reason.

Choice of wrong timing to operate acute cholecystitis is a common cause for surgical difficulties and eventually surgical accidents. There is evidence that performing cholecystectomy more than 5 or 6 days after the onset of the acute inflammation will make surgery much more difficult and face a great number of serious inflammatory adhesions, causing much more bleeding than usual and making it difficult to recognise proper anatomy and surgical landmarks.

Some signs, visible previously to surgery or during it, shall lead to the suspicion that serious inflammation may be present; thick gallbladder wall (>5 mm) at US, firm adherence of gallbladder to omentum, duodenum, colon or stomach, liver pulled down around a shrunken gallbladder or when the surgeon cannot find the gallbladder are some of these.

Before following on to other possible causes, let us summarise patient's ones. One must not forget who the high-risk patients for iatrogenic lesions are:

Male patients
Patients with cirrhosis or liver steatosis
Obese patients
Those having had previous upper abdominal surgeries
Those having delayed treatment of acute cholecystitis

A multitude of technical mishaps are causes for complications, most of them being present due to the ineptitudes of the surgical team and from some of its technical options:

Bad ports positioning, in the case of laparoscopic approach, is an evident cause, but many times these are not properly weighed. By itself, or because of the above, a bad field exposition and bad illumination are also reasons for a higher incidence of complications. Too much smoke or too much blood in the field can hamper visibility to a point of danger.

There is a need to have the ports correctly positioned regarding the possible location of the gallbladder, patient's BMI and configuration and size of the instruments being used.

In the same line, bad anaesthesia is a well-known factor by contributing to bad visualisation of the operating field; patient's lack of relaxation will "close" the operating field.

Surgeon's (or team's) inexperience as well as surgeon's (or team's) tiredness are very often disregarded or not recognised. In connection with these factors is not knowing of eventual anomalies; these anomalies are frequent, well known and defined and represent a serious situation, which, if not recognised, give no excuses to the surgeons involved. No surgeon shall undertake any kind of surgery without minimal theoretical and practical preparation, much more so in the biliary field, where important anomalies are so frequent. On the other hand, also related to "experience", surgeon's overconfidence can be a cause of BDI, by "simplifying" some cases or some technical steps of surgery.

The surgeon can, still, be a cause of BDI, by not paying attention to some crucial points: performing surgery with a bad vision angle, using wrong instruments and applying wrong use of technologies are, too often, causes of lesions.

In a similar level, technical failures come as causes for complications; some of these are surgical technique failures, some instrumental ones. Inappropriate traction of structures, supposedly for "better exposition", can alter the anatomical relations and be a cause of lesions; the same goes for undue use of diathermia, which, unfortunately, we see too often, either by using it too strongly or for too long. Another point for which care is mandatory relates to proper maintenance of instruments; especially reusable ones can have deficient isolation, giving rise to coupling lesions, when, while using electrosurgery, non-visible sparks jump from the instrument to organs away from vision, with consequent thermal lesions.

Instrumental mishaps are, sometimes, unavoidable, but their occurrence must be anticipated, and backup material and/or appropriate maintenance and repair are a must. Instruments can be broken, tipped or sharp pointed, can be inappropriate for the task or can mechanically malfunction.

Let us look at an important point related to these issues: human error. The so called "learning curve", with its associated human error, which is so often used nowadays in surgery as an "explanation" for some complications, would never be accepted in high-technology industries or in some sensitive areas like airlines or military. Many mandatory preparation steps have been designed by these groups to impose rules and protocols, in order to minimise the problems; soon we may have to do the same and follow, for instance, a complete checklist procedure before and during each surgical operation; checklists are a controversial point to be discussed under a different approach. Training, on the other hand, is a capital issue and it is necessary to keep full attention to this sector.

Human errors can happen, nevertheless, despite all efforts to avoid them; we have to minimise them to the extreme. More often, they are based on technical, training or knowledge failures (ignorance) and with non-compliance to established rules. These are the ones "easier" to control. Others are related to a complex and not well-known phenomenon: visual failure or misguidance.

Included amongst processes called "heuristic", human brain can induce visual errors that, no matter what further obvious changes there are in the visual field, become stable and understood as reality, staying like that for the whole surgery. This means that, under certain circumstances, anatomic structures are perceived as different ones in the beginning of the surgery (the most common one being interpreting the CBD as being the cystic duct), and the brain "keeps telling" that this first perception is the correct one, leading to the crucial iatrogenic lesion [8].

In a more practical example, this process can also be called "optical illusion" and is well exemplified in the two drawings below: in one, called the Kanizsa's triangle, half of the viewers will see a black-lined triangle, the other half a white one; the other drawing will show six or seven cubes piled in different directions, again depending on the first view of the observer. As a matter of fact, in Kanizsa's triangle, there is no triangle: just three angles and three "Packman drawings", which, in togetherness, compose the image(s) that the brain "thinks" to be the right one (see Figs. 2.2 and 2.3).

Way and Lawrence have shown in 2003 that the great majority of iatrogenic lesions of the biliary tract (97 %) are caused by errors in visual perception and only 3 % because of technical errors (Fig. 2.4).

This means that most lesions are caused by "intentional" actions by surgeons (not realising it, evidently), leading to unintentional results. These errors of visual perception can be caused – besides the basic problem – by visual difficulties under special situations: inflammation, too much cephalic retraction and, at the same time, insufficient lateral retraction, and "camel hump" position of the CBD because of too much upper traction of the gallbladder infundibulum [9].

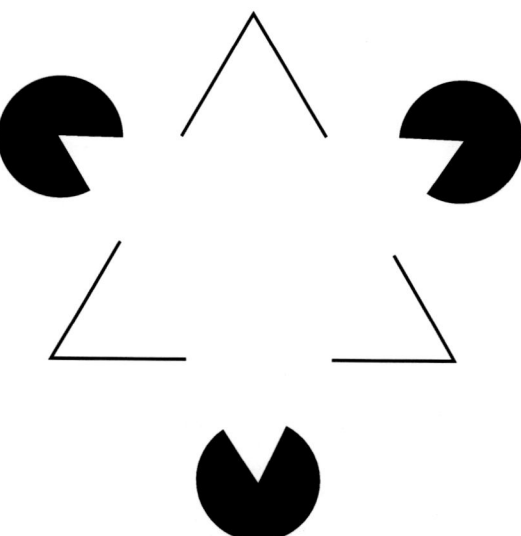

**Fig. 2.2** Kanizsa's triangle

**Fig. 2.3**

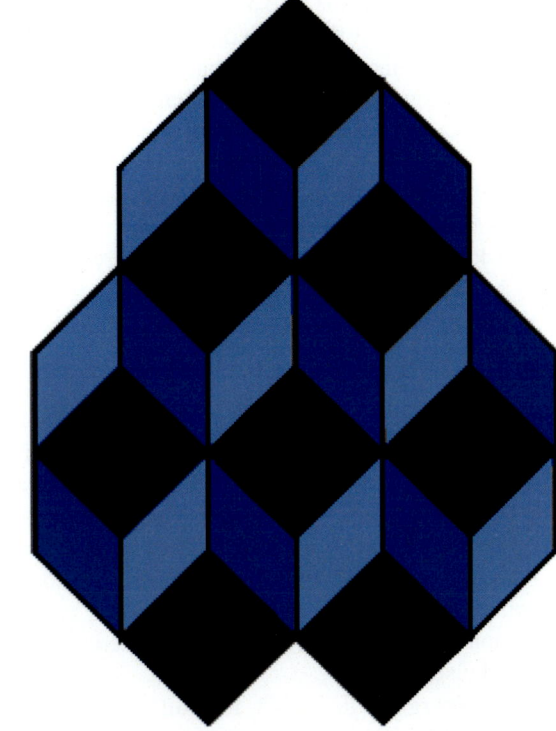

**Fig. 2.4** Rate of technical (3 %) and non-technical (97 %) causes of errors leading to iatrogenic bile lesions

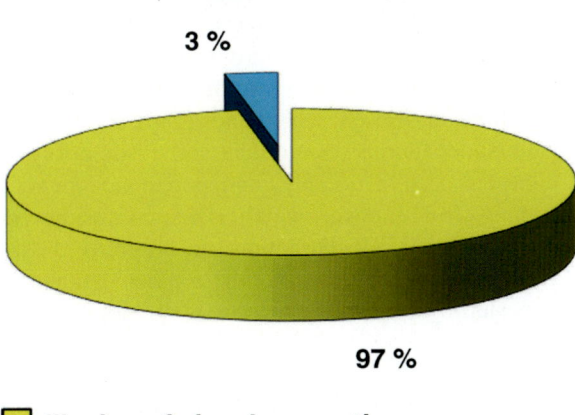

**Illusion of visual perception**

## 2.3   Prevention (with Tips and Tricks)

Many of the explanations for the "causes" are, at the same time, self-explaining regarding what has to be done for "prevention" of the complications.

We can consider that one of the most important issues, which allow minimisation of complications, is correct indication and preparation of patients for any given surgery. Fast-track is also a possibility for these patients, but let us not forget that the whole concept of fast-track does not allow "forgetting" to apply all necessary steps.

All these factors lead to "paradigms of avoidable error", which are a challenge for every surgeon involved in biliary surgery.

The questions and paradigms are:

Can the use of a meticulous technique and of an intense effort to identify the anatomy avoid lesions?

It is known that prosecuting "excellency" can diminish the rate of complications, but can it ever avoid it completely?

Will the results of any working group or surgeon always be conditioned by statistical compilations?

Statistically, it can still be said that, despite all efforts, a lesion of the biliary tract will always occur, at least once during the career of any GI surgeon. Because of this, in the end, and the most important: are complications inevitable??

While the goal should really be minimising harm, this does not seem at the moment completely avoidable. Only a culture of prosecution of quality and excellence, using all means at our disposition and implementing checklists, protocols, compliance of rules and proper training, can lead, eventually, to ground zero of complications. Checklists, as mentioned before, are a subject to be discussed in detail elsewhere.

Strasberg has defended, for quite some time now, that the systematic use of the so-called "Critical View of Safety" (CVS) – his dissection technique – can prevent the occurrence of iatrogenic lesions; in some countries, it is mandatory to use this dissection approach and to provide evidence of its use, the best evidence being provided by images, either video or still photos [10]. CVS dissection consists of performing a dissection, which ends up by showing only two structures coming to the gallbladder fundus (cystic duct and cystic artery) (Fig. 2.5). This dissection technique has been favourably compared to the "funnel" one, also called "infundibular", coming from above, which risks confusion between CBD and cystic duct. Nevertheless, CSV dissection can be pretty difficult to achieve in "the difficult" gallbladder. We believe that these cases demand a much more meticulous dissection, step-by-step until a close to CVS view can be obtained.

## 2.3.1  Lesions of the Biliary Tract

These are the most serious, in general, complications in biliary surgery (as well as in other surgeries, as mentioned in the beginning). Many lines have been written about these lesions, when laparoscopic surgery became widespread, many of them calling attention to the problem and many implying that laparoscopic surgery was the culprit of all of it.

What seems to be true is that these lesions are more severe than the ones existing previously, in the times of "open" cholecystectomy [11].

**Fig. 2.5** On the left can be seen the positioning of clips in a tubular structure, after finishing dissection and before cutting the cystic duct. The photo on the *right side* shows the "Critical View of Safety", in a case where the view could be misleading, with the cystic duct highly implanted. In this case, there was a risk of cutting, inadvertently, the common bile duct

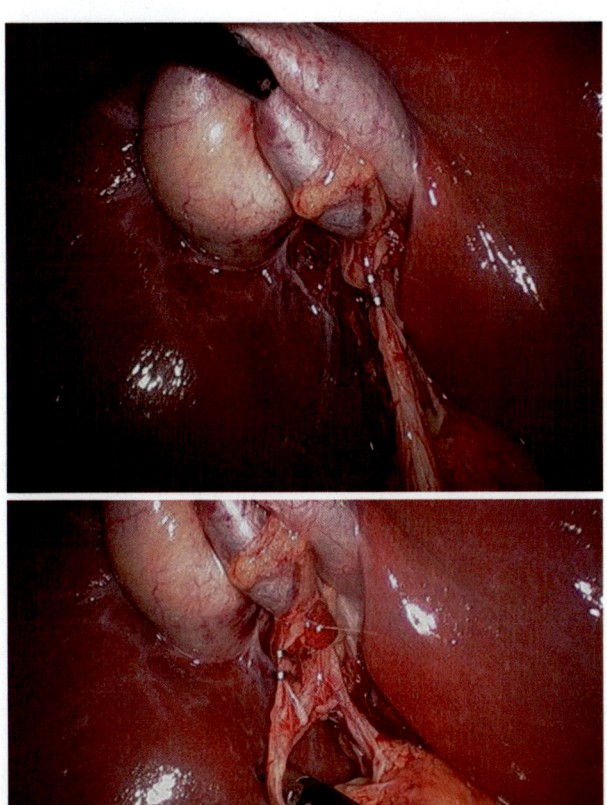

Calling the attention to the problem, already in 1944, Grey Turner wrote in the "Lancet": "CBD lesions are, almost always, a result of an accident during surgery, and, therefore, it can only be attributed to the surgical profession... ...These lesions cannot be seen as a normal operative risk..."

The total rate is not high in global terms, but the real importance relates to the seriousness of these complications, mainly considering that its majority happens during surgery for benign situations (Table 2.2).

Some patients have specific causes for a higher possibility of lesions, either by their own comorbidities or by problems, errors or mistakes during surgery. Compromised healing in patients with bad nutrition status, cachexia or under treatment with steroids or immunosuppressors is one of the possible causes, and it shall be anticipated by the surgeon, before operation, bringing a serious state of alertness. Bactibilia, which may happen in up to 90 % of patients with acute cholecystitis, is

**Table 2.2** Incidence of iatrogenic lesions of biliary tract

| Type of surgery | Study (author) | No. patients | Rate (%) |
|---|---|---|---|
| Laparoscopy | France | 24 300 | 0.27 |
| | USA | 77 600 | 0.6 |
| | Portugal | 14 455 | 0.25 |
| | Italy | 13 718 | 0.24 |
| | Metanalyses | | 0.8–1 |
| | Strasberg et al. [15] | | 2 |
| | Nuzzo et al. [12] | | 0.31 |
| Laparotomy | Johns Hopkins (H. Pitt) | | 0.1–0.2 |
| | San Diego (A. R. Moossa) | | 0.5 |
| | Paul-Brousse (H. Bismuth) | | 0.2 |
| | Cornell Univ. (L. Blumgart) | | 0.2 |
| | Portug. Soc. Surg. (B. Castelo) | | 0.55 |
| | Davidoff et al. [20] | | 0.2 |
| | Nuzzo et al. [12] | | 0.1 |
| Laparoscopy x "classic" | McMahon et al. [22] | Increase of: | 0.5 |
| Laparoscopy x "classic" | Davidoff et al. [19] | Times more | 5–10 |
| "Diminished" | Richardson et al. [21] | Less: | 0.4–0.8 |

another serious risk factor. Others may be cholangitis, gallbladder empyema, jaundice, CBD stones, acute cholecystitis and age above 70 years.

A. R. Moossa very well defined the "3 dangers" regarding the risk of having biliary tract lesions during surgery:

1. Dangerous disease – relating to situations where local surgical conditions convert the "surgical territory" into an area of difficult management because of inflammation, sclerosis, fibrosis or exuberant vascular territory, as it happens in cases of late acute cholecystitis or portal hypertension.
2. Dangerous anatomy – in the cases (about 10–15 %) where there are anatomic anomalies; it is necessary that the surgeon is well aware of the incidence and of the types of anomalies. While some are of no surgical importance, others can lead to catastrophe.
3. Dangerous surgery – although technical deficiencies can happen without warning, some others can be anticipated, and preventive measures can be applied. Surgery performed by surgeons or teams without proper physical or training conditions is another scenario leading to disaster.

Direct causes for biliary stenosis – early and late – are:

1. Tying, cutting or resecting the CBD
2. Luminal occlusion (total or partial, when tying the cystic duct – the "camel hump" situation)
3. Ischemia of CBD (too much dissection can cause this)

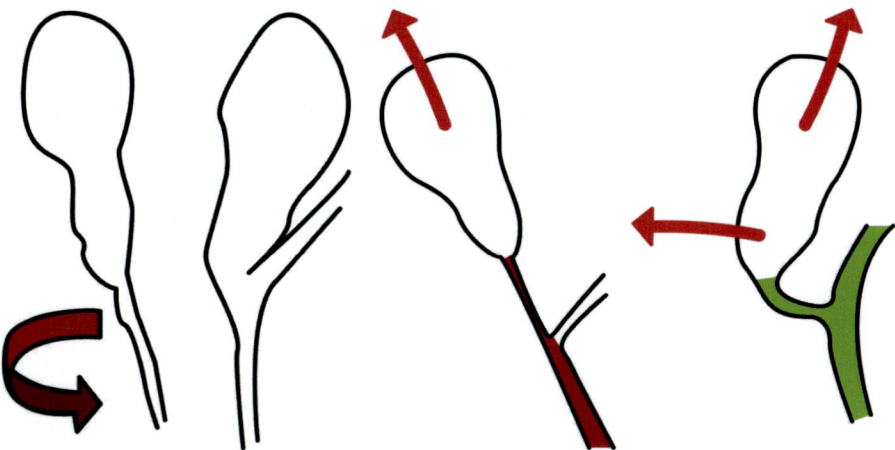

**Fig. 2.6** These drawings show the importance of the execution of the "flagging" manoeuvre and of the proper directions of traction of the fundus and of the infundibulum of the gallbladder. "Flagging" and turning around the infundibulum can show the correct position of the CBD, avoiding the "hiding CBD syndrome", which can be a major cause of a serious lesion (see Video 2.1). On the *right side,* it is shown how correct traction can help: retracting the infundibulum of the gallbladder to the right misaligns the cystic duct from the common bile duct showing clearly which is which

4. Periductal ischemia (same cause)
5. Luminal trauma while exploring
6. (Pre-existing benign stenosis – very rare nowadays)

All of these can happen without the awareness of the surgeon, mainly because of the reasons exposed above. Nevertheless, some measures can be applied before and during surgery, to prevent these lesions:

- Surgical access shall be adapted to morphology – this can happen when a non-routine placement of trocars is used; placement has to be chosen individually, according to the patient's anatomy.
- Good exposure of the hepato/duodenal space – by judicious use of patient's positioning and traction of gallbladder's fundus and neck. A movement with the forceps, forcing a "flag in the flagpole" display of cystic duct's face, right, left and back views, will help in preventing lesions. The same applies to the Critical View of Safety dissection (Fig. 2.6).
- Also, too much traction in the gallbladder neck, and in the wrong direction, can pull the common bile duct from its normal location, causing the so-called "camel hump" position of the CBD at cystic channel insertion, leading to its inadvertent clipping and/or partial removal (Fig. 2.7).
- Good identification of structures, before tying, clipping and cutting – this is one of the most important steps in prevention, as we have mentioned, that only a certain constant rate of anatomical anomalies exist, but, in addition, the brain can

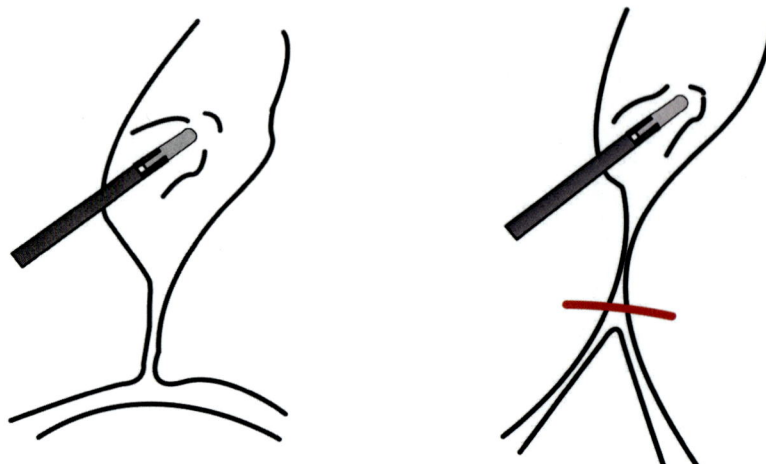

**Fig. 2.7** Traction in the gallbladder, leading to "camel hump" position of the common bile duct; this can cause possible inadvertent clipping of the duct and/or partial removal (see Videos 2.2 and 2.3)

"trick" the vision of the surgical field, inducing perception errors. Using mental checklists for identification of anatomy, with routines in following and showing some portions, and confirming them with the first aide are good measures to diminish this danger.

- Appropriate dissection – follows the same cautions as above and implies the caution of not performing important and irreversible steps in surgery, without being absolutely sure of what is visible; do not "assume" anatomy and structures, and remember that inflammation and fibrosis can hide the correct planes of dissection.
- If necessary, perform direct cholecystectomy – as a safety measure, and this applies for both types of surgery.
- Selective cholangiography – it can be necessary to perform a cholangiography in certain cases, to clarify ductal anatomy; it is necessary to realise that cholangiography implies clipping and cutting the biliary tract and that this action in itself can be the cause of a lesion. The safest way to execute this exam, if one wants to see the anatomy of the biliary tract, is to do it through the gallbladder, before clipping the cystic duct. CBD's puncture for performing the cholangiography can be the cause of postoperative bilomas. Some recent studies show that fluorescence cholangiography can be a very good and non-invasive alternative. As basic understanding, IOC (intraoperative cholangiography) does not avoid, by itself, biliary tract lesions [13].
- Clamping of the pedicle, if big haemorrhage – another important tip; it is imperative, facing difficult bleeding or bleeding which is impossible to control immediately, to have a proper view of the origin of the haemorrhage and to evaluate its amount and possible ways to control it. This can only be done by stopping the

blood flow, and this can be done by means of a clamp in the pedicle. There are ways to do this in laparoscopic surgery, but if the surgeon finds it difficult or too challenging, it is time to either ask for immediate help from someone with higher expertise or to convert. Shooting clips in a blind way to the area where the bleeding seems to come from leads very frequently to serious complications, even if the haemorrhage is controlled.

- The fall of a clip from the cystic artery stump or its inadvertent cutting can, often, lead to a retraction of this stump, with profuse bleeding, behind the hepatic duct. Trying blindly to control this haemorrhage by clips can cause hepatic duct lesions in the area shown in Fig. 2.8.

- Great care with the use of electrosurgery – despite all attention, electrical current follows structures and directions, which the surgeon is often unaware of. Conduction of electricity burns through ductal structures can cause extremely serious and very extensive lesions, sometimes destroying almost the whole extent of the main bile duct. Also, minute problems in the protection layer of certain instruments can give rise to sparks, injuring areas out of sight (the "coupling" problem already mentioned) (see Videos 2.3 and 2.4).

This brings to discussion a question many put:

Are the lesions from laparoscopic surgery more serious?

The fact is, in laparoscopic surgery, some lesions started to show, which did not happen before; these are the lesions caused by total destruction of the CBD, for instance, because of extensive or wrong use of electrosurgery and the ones which imply removal, erroneously, of long lengths of the biliary tract. There has been the implication, by some authors, that some more recent surgical series, regarding

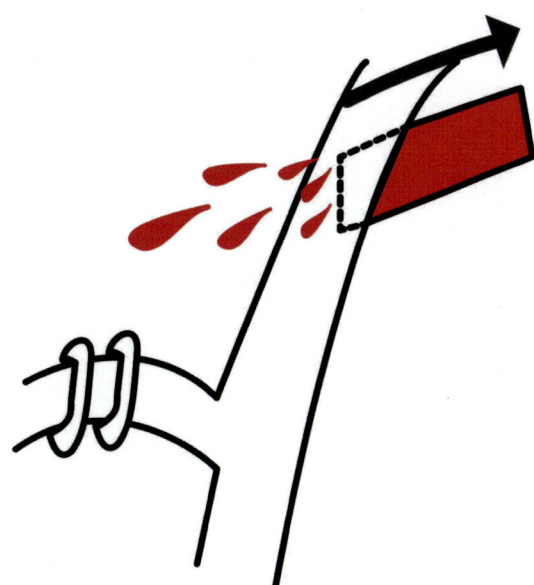

**Fig. 2.8** Artery's retraction behind hepatic duct can be a cause of lesion if the attempts to control it are done blindly

treatment of CBI, have a slightly inferior success rate than older ones; this might be due to the existence of worse lesions in the laparoscopic era. As a matter of fact, about 30 % of lesions, nowadays, are extensive burn lesions. Another type of lesion relates to resection (or excision) of extensive length of the biliary tract. Lesions often very close to the hilum happen a lot as well as their coexistence with biliary fistulae, with consequent increase of inflammation, because of bile action. All these in togetherness with the fact that in many other cases we see bile ducts with small calibre are reasons for the increase of the seriousness of the injuries (Fig. 2.9).

Alternatively, some other lesions are also more benign, like tangential lesions, clip falling or puncture lesions, allowing treatment by minimally aggressive endoscopic methods. Injuries can be graded, from less to more severe, as:

1. Puncture
2. Partial laceration
3. Complete section
4. Obstructing clip
5. Enlarged section (tissue removal)
6. Thermal lesion
7. Thermal necrosis

Some of the less severe can be approached and treated only by endoscopic methods.

More recommendations can be given regarding attitudes to minimise BDI.

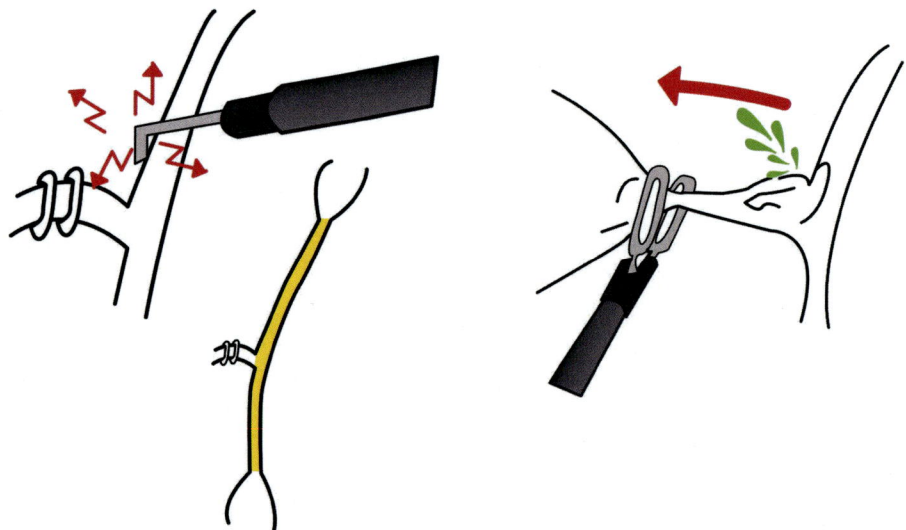

**Fig. 2.9** Thermal lesions cause extensive damage of the bile tract, and rough manipulation can be the reason for large defects of bile ducts (see Video 2.5)

It is necessary for surgeons to keep some technical details in mind, and the permanent use of "prevention" measures, even in the "simplest" surgery setting. Always do a surgical access, adapted to the patient's morphology, giving a good exposure of the hepato/duodenal space and having good identification of structures, before tying or cutting anything. Appropriate dissection and, if necessary, direct cholecystectomy and/or selective cholangiography are another must, as well as a proper clamping of the pedicle if a big haemorrhage is encountered, as means of clear and safe control. Another point is to always maintain great care with the use of electrosurgery. Under certain conditions, dissection of the structures is more hazardous (Fig. 2.10).

As principles to reduce the incidence, one can recommend:

Use of 30° optic.
Use of clear and proper methods for retract and expose to the surgical field.
Dissection of Calot's triangle, starting close to the gallbladder.
Unequivocal identification of cystic duct and artery before they are divided:
Find the cystic duct by starting dissection at the triangle of Calot.
Clear the medial wall of infundibulum.
And trace the cystic duct on an uninterrupted line into the base of the gallbladder.

There are factors that may suggest that the structure being dissected is the CBD, instead of the cystic duct (> Ø duct, course behind duodenum, unexpected duct, large artery, etc.).

Some "principles" have been widely mentioned as rules to prevent lesions. But some may prove wrong:

"Clearly identify the junction of the cystic duct and CBD". Too much dissection work in here can lead to problems such as devascularisation with late strictures.

"Use routine IO cholangiography". Although useful in many situations (confusing anatomy, difficult dissection, anomaly suspected), it brings another possible problem: there is a danger of misinterpretation, giving a false sense of security. The

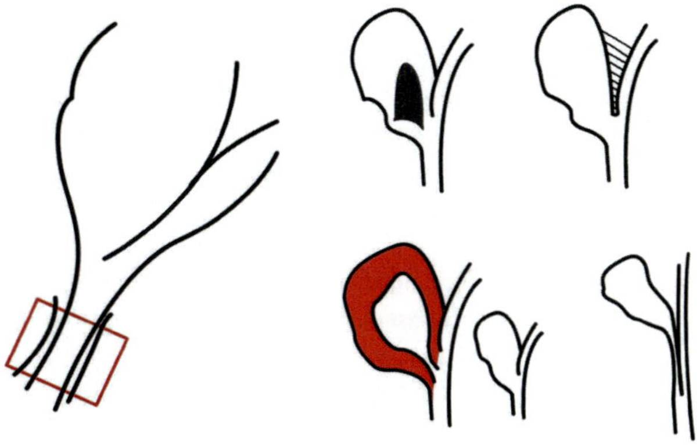

**Fig. 2.10** Ideal dissection area and reasons for this dissection being more difficult: large stone in the infundibulum, extensive local adhesions, acute inflammation and anatomical anomalies

"tricks" the brain does before can also happen with cholangiography. And many lesions happen after cholangiography!

Facing some difficulties, there are options to deal with it:

When a wide cystic duct is found, the surgeon may use 11-mm clips, if available, or use 9 mm at first (it will not close the whole lumen), followed by applying a pre-made endoloop knot.

If many adhesions are present, dissection must stick close to the gallbladder, and special care regarding electrosurgery has to be considered; minimise using monopolar diathermy as much as you can.

With a big stone in the Hartman pouch, there are ways to move it out of the way, simplifying dissection: try to move the stone up and grasp the Hartman below it.

Or use a lateral grasper for retracting the liver, without holding the fundus. The other two graspers manipulate the stone up. If this fails, try to support the Hartman by a grasper, and dissect the Calot's triangle. Again, if this fails, open the Hartman pouch, and extract the stone.

When the left lobe of the liver encroaches the operative field, making visualisation difficult, raise the right shoulder of the patient, or use a long port or retractor from the epigastric incision. The surgeon can also retract the fundus upwards and medially. Finally, one may put a port more to retract the left lobe.

In some cases, the gallbladder is difficult to grasp; it is necessary to empty the GB totally or partially.

Anytime a surgeon considers that an anomaly may exist, one of three solutions shall be used:

- Intraoperative cholangiography (properly interpreted)
- Getting a second opinion (presence of the help in the OT)
- Convert

## 2.4 Main Dissection Techniques

There are two main techniques to execute laparoscopic cholecystectomy:

1) The infundibular technique [14]. In this technique, the surgeon is taught to clear the infundibulum of the gallbladder (bowl of a funnel) down to the cystic duct (stem of the funnel) all the way around 360°.

   Supposedly, when the funnel is seen, the cystic duct is identified.

2) The Critical View of Safety approach [15–17] which was mentioned before, and which is based on the fact that it is considered to have a safe and clear anatomy to finish surgery only when nothing else than two structures are visible coming out of the gallbladder. CVS (Critical View of Safety) is not really a dissection method; it is more a safety identification approach. It was first described in 1992 but only called as CVS in 1995 [15–17].

When approaching the gallbladder, it is necessary to remember that "biliary inflammation fusion" sticks anatomical elements together and makes it difficult to find where one structure starts and another ends. It makes the cystic duct look like the CBD and can change an "easy" cholecystectomy into a "difficult" one.

CVS has, as its true value, minimisation of risks. Using this approach, surgeon's limit for conversion becomes lower or increases the possibility of using ancillary techniques like intraoperative cholangiography to better evaluate the picture, minimising risks (see Videos 2.1, 2.2 and 2.3).

Steven Strasberg [15, 18] is very critical of infundibular approach and considers it as an "error trap", when trying to identify the cystic duct. His reasoning is that, the funnel shape, which is necessary to obtain the correct view, may, sometimes, be obtained by the dissection itself, and the stem of this funnel is not the cystic duct; this is because, in this technique, the surgeon is taught to clear the infundibulum of the gallbladder (bowl of a funnel) down to the cystic duct (stem of the funnel) all the way around 360°. Supposedly, when the funnel is seen, the cystic duct is identified. If the view is obtained by the dissection, the error is there, and another structure other than the cystic duct is cut.

The basis of CVS consists in three fundamental steps: no fibrotic tissue or fat at the Calot's triangle, freeing the lower third of the gallbladder from its bed and checking the two structures (only two) coming into the gallbladder.

Finally, which suggestions and recommendations on measures to minimise the problem can be given?

Mainly two: following guidelines and improving training and education. Some guidelines are well established and have good grades of recommendation: optimal exposure to reach the Critical View of Safety is highly recommended (GoR B). Although this can be achieved with the 0°, 30° or 45° optics, the CBD is more difficult to see with the 0° because it lies parallel to the scope. Rotation of the angled scopes provides different visualisation of the surgical field. This was already proposed long ago [16].

Inability to reach the Critical View of Safety and/or to identify the source and safely control bleeding, are indications for conversion (GoR A).

It is recommended to have supervised structured training, starting with skills courses (GoR B).

In some countries, it is mandatory to have a routine demonstration that CVS was obtained, either by photos or by video recording [16, 17].

Clearly, although BDI do occur in the hands of expert surgeons, inadequate experience is a risk factor.

New educational methods shall be put into practice, and already enough experience exists to understand this. Besides known exercises and properly structured courses, some more recent ideas have been understood. Expert surgeons can be identified, and their techniques have to be put in practice in teaching methods; they must share their practical preventing measures. This may bring learners faster to the level of "experts".

Experts have more knowledge and, consequently, superior performance, although some of the reasons for this cannot be clearly understood; the most important is called "hidden knowledge". This has three types:

Informal knowledge – from experience, but unwritten: does not exist in textbooks. An example is something many have experienced: the expert tells the resident to stop and look "here" or "there". Looking, one finds that there was a reason for that. But all the expert can say is "It just didn't look right".

Impressionistic knowledge – experts are always, even unconsciously, looking back into "past experiences". They have some "impressions" of some situations, with a "feeling of possible danger" in the presence of certain signs, not described.

Self-regulation knowledge – deep knowledge about themselves and about how they act.

Other evident but not so often followed principles – these can be generalised for any surgical approach – are the constant use of the highest human and surgical good sense, as well as keeping an adequate knowledge of the anatomy, and of the anomalies. Last, but by no means least, whenever in doubt, stop and re-evaluate; one will be surprised by the number of times this will change the options and attitudes. And always keep a humble position; be aware of the situations and of the capacities, human and technical, existing. Every time it feels advisable, do not hesitate to ask for help.

As general conclusions, it can be said that these are serious lesions. They can be avoided (or at least, minimised), by a cautious approach, a surgeon's liberal policy of conversion and asking for specialised help when facing unexpected intraoperative problems. No surgeon is "protected" against this problem, and correct training in laparoscopy is mandatory. These lesions, by their specificity, should always be dealt with by experienced teams in reference centres. Only this way, complications can be minimised and quality and good outcomes guaranteed.

# References

1. Morgenstern L, Berci G (1992) Twelve hundred open cholecystectomies before the laparoscopic era a standard for comparison leon. Arch Surg 127(4):400–403
2. Castelo B et al (1998) Portug Soc Surg. Personal communication.
3. Chapman WC et al (1995) Postcholecystectomy bile duct strictures. Management and outcome in 130 patients. Arch Surg 130(6):597–602; discussion 602–604
4. Maetani Y, Itoh K et al (1998) Portal vein anomaly associated with deviation of the ligamentum teres to the right and malposition of the gallbladder. Radiology 207(3):723–728
5. Voitk AJ, Tsao SG et al (2001) The tail of the learning curve for laparoscopic cholecystectomy. Am J Surg 182(3):250–253
6. Morgenstern L. McGrath MF et al (1995) Continuing hazards of the learning curve in laparoscopic cholecystectomy. Am Surg 61(10):914–918
7. Calvete J, Sabater L et al (2000) Bile duct injury during laparoscopic cholecystectomy: myth or reality of the learning curve? Surg Endosc 14(7):608–611
8. Way LW et al (2003) Causes and prevention of laparoscopic bile duct injuries: analysis of 252 cases from a human factors and cognitive psychology perspective. Ann Surg 237(4):460–469
9. Fullum TM et al (2013) Is Laparoscopy a Risk Factor for Bile Duct Injury During Cholecystectomy?. JSLS 17(3):365–370
10. Buddingh KT et al (2012) Documenting correct assessment of biliary anatomy during laparoscopic cholecystectomy. Surg Endosc 26(1):79–85

11. McPartland KJ, Pomposelli JJ (2008) Iatrogenic biliary injuries: classification, identification, and management. Surg Clin North Am 88(6):1329–1343; ix. doi:10.1016/j.suc.2008.07.006
12. Nuzzo G (2009) Treatment of biliary lesions due to cholecystectomy. Chir Ital 61(5–6): 519–521
13. Slim K, Martin G (2013) Does routine intra-operative cholangiography reduce the risk of biliary injury during laparoscopic cholecystectomy? An evidence-based approach. J Visc Surg 150(5):321–324
14. Hunter JG (1991) Avoidance of bile duct injury during laparoscopic cholecystectomy. Am J Surg 162(1):71–76
15. Strasberg SM, Hertl M et al (1995) An analysis of the problem of biliary injury during laparoscopic cholecystectomy. J Am Coll Surg 180(1):101–125
16. Buddingh TK et al (2011) Intraoperative assessment of biliary anatomy for prevention of bile duct injury: a review of current and future patient safety interventions. Surg Endosc 25: 2449–2461
17. Rawlings A et al (2010) Single-Incision Laparoscopic Cholecystectomy: Initial Experience with Critical View of Safety Dissection and Routine Intraoperative Cholangiography. J Am Coll Surg 211(1):1–7
18. Strasberg SM (2013) A teaching program for the "culture of safety in cholecystectomy" and avoidance of bile duct injury. J Am Coll Surg 217(4):751
19. Davidoff AM, Pappas TN et al (1992) Mechanisms of major biliary injury during laparoscopic cholecystectomy. Ann Surg 215(3):196–202
20. Davidoff AM, Branum GD et al (1993) Clinical features and mechanisms of major laparoscopic biliary injury. Semin Ultrasound CT MR 14(5):338–345
21. Richardson MC, Bell G et al (1996) Incidence and nature of bile duct injuries following laparoscopic cholecystectomy: an audit of 5913 cases. West of Scotland Laparoscopic Cholecystectomy Audit Group. Br J Surg 83(10):1356–1360
22. McMahon AJ, Baxter JN et al (1993) Preventing complications of laparoscopy. Br J Surg 80(12):1593–1594

# Complication in Laparoscopic GERD: A Guide to Prevention and Management

**3**

Cavit Avci

## 3.1 Introduction

Gastro-oesophageal reflux disease (GERD) is one of the most frequent benign disorders of the upper gastrointestinal tract and has a high prevalence in western countries.

GERD is the failure of the anti-reflux barrier, allowing abnormal reflux of gastric contents into the oesophagus, which causes different symptoms and complications.

It is a mechanical disorder, caused by a defective lower oesophageal sphincter (LES). The European Association of Endoscopic Surgery (EAES) [1] has evaluated 18,490 articles to establish current guidelines in the consensus development conference in 2013. According to the report of this conference, surgery is a successful therapeutic option, in well-selected patients, instead of long-term medical treatment that is purely symptomatic.

The goal of the surgical treatment for GERD is to restore this defective zone and create a new barrier to prevent gastro-oesophageal reflux.

The aim is to decrease the reflux symptoms, curing the oesophagitis and improving quality of life by the creation of a new anatomical high-pressure zone. This must be achieved without dysphagia.

The main anti-reflux surgical procedures are based on the wrapping posteriorly of the gastric fundus, total or partial, around the oesophagus, obtaining a new valve able to contrast the reflux when the stomach is full and to adequately relax during swallowing, preventing postoperative dysphagia.

**Electronic supplementary material** The online version of this chapter (doi:10.1007/978-3-319-19623-7_3) contains supplementary material, which is available to authorized users.

C. Avci, MD
General and Laparoscopic Surgery, Istanbul University Medical School, Istanbul, Turkey
e-mail: cavitavci@gmail.com

© Springer International Publishing Switzerland 2016
C. Avci, J.M. Schiappa (eds.), *Complications in Laparoscopic Surgery:
A Guide to Prevention and Management*, DOI 10.1007/978-3-319-19623-7_3

Rudolph Nissen [2] was the first to pioneer anti-reflux surgery in 1956. Although his first approach, 360° fundoplication procedure, improved reflux symptoms, some patients were troubled by dysphagia, bloating and the inability to belch "gas-bloat syndrome." To avoid these side effects, in 1963 André Toupet [3, 4] created a posterior partial (270°) fundoplication, and Belsey [5] and Hill [6] would follow in 1967, with their approaches aimed at restoring the normal physiology of the lower oesophageal sphincter (LES). Subsequently, Mario Rossetti [7] proposed in 1977 a revision that included a modified total fundoplication with minimal dissection of the cardia and no division of the short gastric vessels (SGVs). DeMeester [8] published his "floppy Nissen modification" and successful outcomes in 1986. It concerned a very short 360° fundoplication in a tension-free manner by dividing the short gastric vessels.

More than three decades after the original fundoplication technique which was described by Rudolf Nissen, the first laparoscopic anti-reflux interventions that are based on the creation of a new valve with gastric fundus around the oesophagus, able to contrast the reflux, was described by Bernard Dallemagne in 1991 [9–11].

Since the first laparoscopic anti-reflux procedures, surgical techniques have gradually become standardised and have ended up being the "gold standard" for the treatment of gastro-oesophageal reflux.

Nowadays, laparoscopic anti-reflux surgery is the treatment of choice for patients with recurrent symptoms after suspension of the medication, poor responders to PPI and those not compliant to a long and expensive medical therapy (especially young patients).

Today all types of fundoplication can be carried out in good conditions for well-selected patients, in accordance with well-defined rules. However, surgery is burdened by some complications, side effects and non-negligible reintervention rates [12].

## 3.2 Complications in GERD

### 3.2.1 Generality

Surgical complications of laparoscopic techniques for GERD are generally rare and due to non-compliance with well-codified rules. Certainly, lack of experience of the operator is one of the main risk factors for complications [13]. At the beginning, during the first learning phase, the main difficulty resided in the dissection of the oesophageal hiatus, particularly of the posterior surface of the oesophagus, where the appearance of a certain number of complications, even intra-operative perforations were common.

Progressively, better standardisation and understanding of the laparoscopic view and management of the hiatal region, including dissection in contact with the pillars of the diaphragm, the distance to the oesophagus, the development of instruments for laparoscopic surgery, as well as the appearance of teams with experience have allowed to reproduce techniques, with fewer complications, and more effectively.

**Table 3.1** Complication rate of the multicentre study of the SFCL (French Society of Laparoscopic Surgery) in 1994 [15] and of the series of Dallemagne [16] in 1995

| Authors | Number of cases | Morbidity (%) | Mortality (%) |
|---|---|---|---|
| Champault (1994) FDCL | 940 | 5 | 0.3 |
| Dallemagne (1995) (compilation) | 2149 | 1.6 (reinterventions) | |

Complication rate is often higher at the beginning of the experience, but, in general, it will stabilise after 50 procedures performed by a team and after 20 individual operations per surgeon [14].

Complications of laparoscopic treatment of GERD are the incidents that occur during intervention or the ones that appear during the postoperative course. They are related to the technique, to the experience, to the instrumentation and terrain, etc. and can be of two kinds:

- *Intra-operative complications* (minor or serious)
- *Postoperative complications (failures)* (immediate or delayed)

## 3.2.2 Intra-operative Complications

Intra-operative complications of laparoscopic anti-reflux procedures are essentially traumatic and involve mainly the oesophagus, stomach, pleura and vessels.

As shown in Table 3.1, the publication of Champault [15] related to a multicentre study by the SFCL (French Society of Laparoscopic Surgery) in 1994, the morbidity rate was 5 % with 940 cases of anti-reflux surgery, and in the series of Dallemagne [16] in 1995, with 2149 cases, the complication rate was addressed 1.6 %.

## 3.2.3 Complications/Multicentre Series

Another most recent multicentre study of 7531 patients operated on between 2005 and 2009 shows a 3.8 % morbidity and 0.19 % mortality [17].

Intra-operative complications can be classified into three main groups:

- *Bleeding-haemorrhage*
- *Perforation (oesophagus, stomach)*
- *Other* (pneumothorax-capnothorax, pneumomediastinum-capnomediastinum, laceration, injury or ischaemia in surrounding tissues or organs – liver, stomach, spleen, etc.

### 3.2.3.1 Haemorrhage
Haemorrhagic complications are rarely reported in literature. The overall rate of bleeding is low and usually without vital impact (rare cause of conversion and of transfusions).

Sometimes the type of intervention favours the bleeding. Dissection and section of the short gastric vessels during Nissen's operation may cause injury of the spleen or short vessels (Video 3.1). Nissen-Rossetti, Toupet or Hill's techniques do not seem to cause this type of injury. One of the major bleeding complications is the serious injury of the spleen; this, fortunately, is exceptional in laparoscopic surgery, while, on the contrary, it was quite common during open surgery [15].

A wound of the vena cava inferior or aorta can cause a very severe haemorrhagic accident; this may occur during the dissection of mediastinal oesophagus, during suturing of the diaphragmatic crus or when attaching a prosthesis on the hiatal defect. Be careful.

Otherwise, no significant bleeding from wounds in relatively small vessels or the liver injury by the retractor can often occur without serious consequences and are, often, stopped with a simple coagulation or ligation (Video 3.2).

Contrary to this, recklessly cutting a large left hepatic artery without effective haemostasis can be a cause of serious bleeding (Video 3.3). In the case of a large artery, effective control with ligatures, clips or LigaSure or ultrasonic dissection should be absolutely made before the section.

Video 3.1: Haemorrhage short gastric vessels
Video 3.2: Bleeding from relatively small vessels
Video 3.3: Serious haemorrhage during inattentive dissection of the lesser curvature

### 3.2.3.2 Digestive Perforations

Digestive Intra-operative complications are primarily represented by perforation of hollow organs (oesophagus and stomach). These complications were rarely mentioned in open series and seem to be rather specific of laparoscopy.

The series of the first years, in the beginning of laparoscopic GERD treatment, some cases of gastrointestinal perforation were published. With increasing experience and because of other reasons, these serious complications are rarely described in the most recent series.

In a survey by the French Association of Surgery, from 1999 [18] which includes 2424 cases from 21 centres, 25 gastrointestinal perforations were reported; 13 are perforations of the oesophagus and 12 of the stomach, with the need for 5 major surgeries and 2 deaths. Champault [15] has reported eight perforations in the research done by the FDCL, in 1994. Hinder [19] has reported 20 cases in 2453 patients. These perforations are estimated to be around 1 % and are quite serious as they are responsible for the majority of deaths reported in those series.

There is a classic mechanism to cause these wounds of the oesophagus and stomach:

• Peri-oesophagitis with the cardia fixed in the lower mediastinum
• The brachy-oesophagus;
• Reoperations

**Table 3.2**  Complications/wounds of the oesophagus, in the AFC study [18]

|  | Intra-operative diagnosis – 9 |  |  |  |
|---|---|---|---|---|
| Intervention | Conversion | Laparoscopic suturing | No problems |  |
| 8 FC, 1 FP | 6 | 3 | 3 |  |
|  | Postoperative diagnosis – 4 |  |  |  |
| Intervention | Time to diagnosis | Reintervention | No problems | Death |
| 3 FC, 1 Ang | 1–25 days | 4 | 3 | 1 |

- Bad dissection plane with forceful passing behind the oesophagus
- Perforation during passage of the tube (Faucher or other)
- Electrical lesions of the oesophagus
- Aggressive use of the instruments
- Perforation by dropping stitches
- Large hiatal hernia
- Obesity

### 3.2.3.3 Oesophageal Perforation

Oesophageal perforation is the most important complication of anti-reflux surgery. It represents 0–2 % of cases depending on the series, occurring mainly during the phase of retro-esophageal hiatal dissection region. The consequence varies and can be detected early or late. If it is discovered during the operation, it has the chance to repair perhaps laparoscopically and during recovery. Otherwise, unknown oesophageal perforation may result a severe complication, even death.

In the investigation of the AFC [18], 13 oesophageal perforations have been reported, and 9 were diagnosed intraoperatively, requiring 6 times a conversion. The diagnosis of the other four cases is done within 1–25 days. In 12 cases, the suites were simples. One death has been reported in a patient of 48 years, operated for a complete fundoplication, and, in which the removal of the valve was made by thoracic approach. All oesophageal wounds were sutured, three laparoscopically. A wound of the oesophagus occurred during the passage of tube Faucher (Table 3.2).

*Prevention*: Especially when there is the higher risk of oesophageal perforation, this can be minimised by the way retro-oesophageal dissection is performed, remaining in contact with the pillars of the diaphragm.

To avoid puncturing the oesophagus, we must not forget the basic principles of anti-reflux surgery: "Dissection of the oesophageal hiatus and not of the oesophagus". Most importantly, do pay lots of attention to not let go unnoticed any possible injury, in order to not run the risk of a complication that can be catastrophic.

### 3.2.3.4 Gastric Perforation

Gastric perforations are rarer than oesophagus's. Literature reports a certain number of cases. The series of Watson [20] reports 1 case out of 200, the series of Champault [15] reports 2 cases out of 940 and Hinder's reports 5 cases out of 2453 [19].

**Table 3.3** Complications/gastric wounds, in the series of the AFC [18]

|              | Intra-operative diagnosis – 3 |                       |                           |                         |       |
|--------------|-------------------------------|-----------------------|---------------------------|-------------------------|-------|
| Intervention | Conversion                    | Laparoscopic suturing | No problems               | Reintervention          | Death |
| 2 FC, 1 FP   | 2                             | 1                     | 2                         | 1 gastrectomy           | 0     |
|              | Postoperative diagnosis – 9   |                       |                           |                         |       |
| Intervention | Time to diagnosis             | Laparoscopic suturing | Laparotomy + thoracotomy  | Iterative intervention  | Death |
| 8 FC, 1 FP   | 1–15 days                     | 1 (day 2)             | 8 (5 sutures, 3 gastrectomies) | 1 oesophageal stenosis | 1     |

In AFC's [18] series, of the 12 gastric wounds reported 3 were pre-operatively discovered and treated; two with sutures and one by a secondary gastrectomy. Nine were postoperatively found, with two necrosis. Six suturing repair and three gastrectomies were performed. One death has been reported in connection with this complication (Table 3.3).

### 3.2.3.5 Complications: Gastric Wounds

Usually the location is anterior, near the greater curvature. Rarely, it is torn by excessive tension of the valve. In this case, the location can be posterior on the valve, retro-oesophageal, close to the pillars. It can also happen as a perforation of the gastric fundus during the difficult dissection in complicated interventions REDO (Video 3.4).

Video 3.4: Gastric perforation of the fundus, during dissection in a REDO surgery

Other rare event of perforation has been described, on the large gastric tuberosity, because of rough use of traumatic forceps. This type of perforation is easier to recognise and can, often, be repaired by laparoscopy [21]. It is also reported in literature, the ischaemic perforation of the great tuberosity due to extensive gastrolysis. Excessive section of short vessels can lead to shortness of blood supply to the great tuberosity relying on the posterior gastric artery whose anatomical variability does not provide for sufficient substitution vessels [22].

### 3.2.3.6 "Gaseous" Complications

Gaseous complications are represented by the pneumothorax and the pneumomediastinum.

The pneumomediastinum is a specific complication of any laparoscopic surgery with opening of the lower mediastinum (GERD, Heller, vagotomy, etc.). Most often it is also because, during this extensive dissection, there was an association with high abdominal pressure. But all patients with dissection pushed into the lower mediastinum and in whom there is high abdominal pressure do not have, systematically, a pneumomediastinum. This mechanism is not the only cause to explain the pneumomediastinum. Perhaps there is an anatomical reason?

The pneumothorax is defined by the passage of $CO_2$ into the pleural cavity through a pleural breach. It is not always the result of the operative act. Decreased oxygen saturation, increased airway pressure and, in particular, abnormal movement of the hemidiaphragm can be called signs of pneumothorax. The diagnosis is made by the analysis of the pleural gas where $CO_2$ can be found.

Joris [23] noted that a capnothorax can be bilateral. Usually, it is well tolerated but it should be treated early. Finally, he showed that PEEP is the most efficient treatment, while it is contraindicated in pneumothorax.

These complications are, in fact, very frequent and less serious.

Pneumothorax requires:

- A pleuropulmonary breach during surgery
- A rupture of an emphysema bullous by increased pressure in the airways

Pleural wounds most often affect the left pleura. The main mechanism is the extensive dissection in the lower part of the mediastinum and going through the wrong retro-oesophageal plan during the dissection of the left side (Video 3.5).

Video 3.5: Pleural wound during mediastinal dissection

### 3.2.3.7 Other Complications

Some anecdotal complications are increasingly reported:

- Cardiac dysrhythmia attributed to a direct myocardial injury [24]
- Acute myopericarditis mechanism [25]
- Cardiac tamponade by wound in the right ventricle [26]

Some specific technical complications have been published in the literature, as some cases of splenic infarction (3 %) (Video 3.6) or very rare cases of necrosis of the gastric valve (0–0.5 %) after section of the short vessels during a Nissen [27–29].

Video 3.6: Partial splenic infarction

## 3.3    Guide to Prevention and Management of Intra-operative Complications

Prevention of complications is the best treatment. Only perfect planning and excellent execution of the technique can minimise complications and their sequelae.

Surgical complications of laparoscopic techniques for GERD are, in general, due to non-compliance with well-standardised surgical steps.

The risk of complications and failure may decrease considerably if there is:

- A correct indication
- Good choice of techniques
- The respect for surgical principles and well-standardised rules

For this reason, we describe, step by step, a classical laparoscopic Nissen operation, emphasising basic principles of anti-reflux surgery and identifying critical technical points.

## 3.3.1   Operating Phases of the Typical Anti-reflux Surgery

Step-1: Dissection of the gastro-oesophageal junction
Step-2: Dissection and mobilisation of the oesophagus
Step-3: Preparation and mobilisation of the gastric fundus
Step-4. Approximation of diaphragmatic pillars (cruroplasty)
Step-5: Creation of the fundus valve (fundoplication)

### 3.3.1.1 Step-1: Dissection of the Gastro-Oesophageal Junction

**Best Exposure of Hiatal Area**
First step of the intervention is to have a good exposure in the hiatal region; for this, a liver retractor is used to lift the left lobe of the liver in order to get a broad view and a perfect exposure.

*Remark*: For work in the hiatal region, to have a good liver retractor is indispensable. The choice of the retractor and its good handling is important. During surgery, a mechanical arm fixed to the right of the operating table, in order to get long-time stability, can hold it.

*Risk*: Liver haemorrhage

*Mechanism:* Inappropriate retractor, careless use

*Prevention:* Select a special atraumatic retractor for the liver, place it carefully and monitor the position during surgery (Fig. 3.1).

**Best Position of the Working Area**
After having installed the liver retractor and obtained a correct working area, the assistant seizes the stomach under the oeso-gastric junction with a grasper and pulls it down and to the left. The gastro-oesophageal junction should remain tense by the pull on that forceps for the security and efficiency of the dissection.

*Remark*: The caudal and leftwards traction of cardia with an atraumatic and appropriate grasper is essential to effective work.

*Risk*: Laceration or even perforation of the stomach.

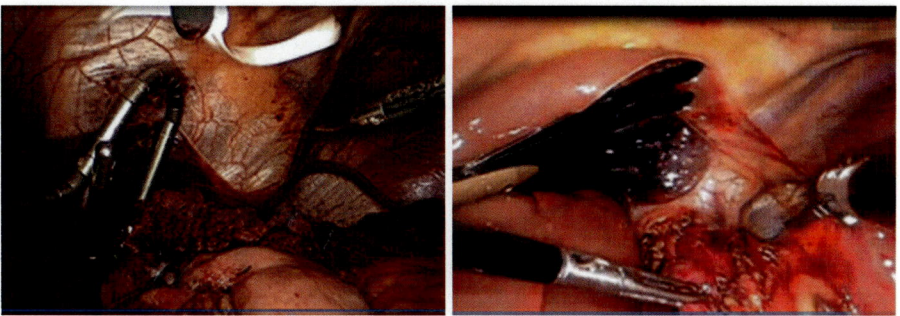

**Fig. 3.1** Two different types of liver retractors

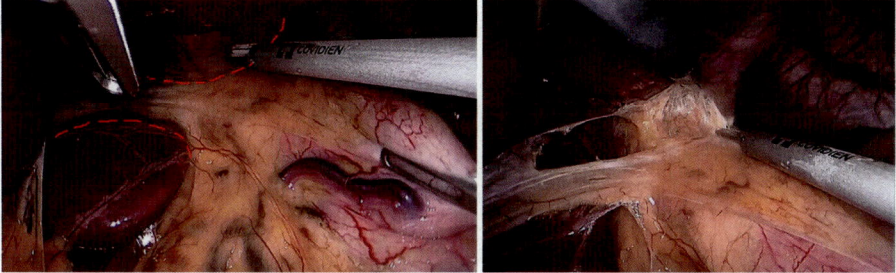

**Fig. 3.2** The large size of the left hepatic artery vagus nerve are preserved

*Mechanism:* Use a traumatic grasper and pull excessively and without care and attention.

*Prevention*: Use only an atraumatic grasper to hold on the cardia and draw up the necessary requirements.

### Opening of the Lesser Omentum and Access to the Right Crus

After good exposure, the lesser omentum is to be sectioned, to allow access to the right crus of the diaphragm. The pars flaccida and pars condensa of the lesser omentum are incised by, at the same time, targeting the upper part of the right crus, which is an essential referral point, before addressing the dissection of the back part of the oesophagus. It is, often, under question whether to preserve or to cut the left hepatic artery which, often, accompanies a left hepatic vagus nerve (Fig. 3.2).

*Remark;* These branches of artery and nerve pass horizontally in the middle of the working field and divide it in two compartments. If it is not cut, working through the upper or lower window of this space will not be very easy.

*Recommendation:* It is recommended, if possible, to preserve a big size artery, without cutting it, even if it makes the approach to the area difficult. If it does not seem very important, this slim branch in the omentum may be cut between two points of haemostasis in order to have suitable working fields. Conversely, if there is an artery of big size, it is advisable not to cut it, even if it makes the approach to

**Fig. 3.3** Dissection of the large-sized lipoma at the hiatus

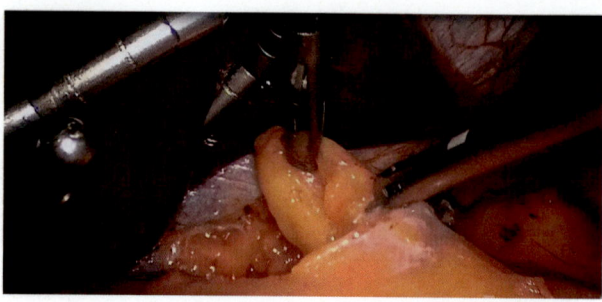

the hiatus harder. In the case of a very thin patient, this is not a problem, but, sometimes, in more obese patients, it is hard to find the crus; so, maybe it is quite helpful to look from below. Meanwhile, this window must be large enough just to admit the fundoplication wrap.

*Risk*: Section of a large artery without effective haemostasis may be a cause of important bleeding (Video 3.2).

*Prevention*: If the left hepatic artery is large, it must be, effectively controlled, with ligatures, clips or proper devices as LigaSure or Ultrasonic Dissector.

### Access the Cardio-oesophageal Junction

The dissection of the cardio-oesophageal junction begins by opening the peritoneal layer of the phreno-oesophageal ligament at the base of the right crus and extends upwardly at its inner edge. This step allows to identify the essential structures: the crura, the vagus nerves, the abdominal part of oesophagus, the mediastinal pleura, the VCI and the aorta.

*Remark:* In some cases, it can show the existence of an annoyingly and significantly sized lipoma at the hiatus; this can make dissection difficult.

Dissection extending up to the inner edge of the crus must not damage the peritoneum covering it, in order to preserve its strength during subsequent rapprochement of the pillars.

*Risk:* The existence of a significantly sized lipoma can prevent the making of a proper fundoplication and can lead to annoying postoperative dysphagia.

Inattentive and deep dissection on the pillars can damage the muscle sheath. This will be a factor in the weakness of the cruroraphy and may lead to postoperative tearing with recurrence of the situation.

*Prevention:* If the size of the hiatal lipoma is important, it is advisable to resect it at the beginning of the dissection; this will allow easy dissection, the creation of a correct fundoplication and the avoidance of an eventual dysphagia after surgery (Fig. 3.3).

Dissection gestures on the pillars must be superficial in order for the sheath of the pillar muscles to remain intact.

### Dissection of the Phreno-oesophageal Ligament

The upper part of the phreno-oesophageal membrane is to be opened transversely, from right to left until the left crus. The dissection can individualise the right edge of the oesophagus and the posterior vagus nerve.

**Figs. 3.4, 3.5, and 3.6**
Dissection and
mobilisation of the
oesophagus

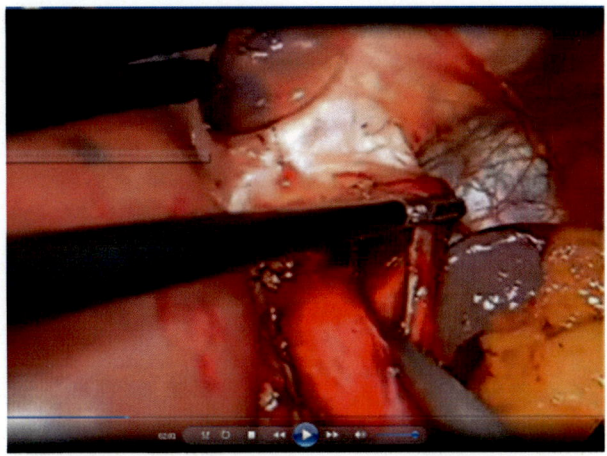

*Remark*: In this step, a blunt dissection, the verification trunks of anterior and posterior vagus nerve is recommended.

Risk: Injury of the oesophageal layer, perforation or section of the vagus nerve.

*Prevention:* This liberation should be very careful and divide the superficial layer of the phreno-oesophageal ligament to avoid injury to some structures at the anterior aspect of the oesophagus, such as the vagus trunk.

### 3.3.1.2 Step-2: Dissection and Mobilisation of the Oesophagus

An incision of the phreno-oesophageal membrane is continued on the medial relief of the right crus, from right to left. The section of the upper part of the gastrophrenic ligament, along the left crus, facilitates the next step (Fig. 3.4). Dissection progresses from inside to outside in front of the left crus until the upper pole of the spleen is identified (Fig. 3.5).

A tape is passed around the oesophago-gastric junction. The traction towards the bottom and outside will help to dissect the lower part of the oesophagus. The dissection around the oesophagus continues into the mediastinum (Fig. 3.6).

*Recommendation*: The left crus must be released as far as possible in order to create an appropriate retro-oesophageal passage; this needs to be wide enough to allow subsequent passage of the anti-reflux valve.

Lifting the gastro-oesophageal junction with a tape allows avoidance of any traumatic grasping of the organs and helps mobilisation of the gastro-oesophageal junction in different directions. It also serves as a landmark to assess the oesophageal segment length below the diaphragm.

Mobilisation of the lower oesophagus must be over a length of 5–10 cm for having an infra-diaphragmatic oesophageal segment length of 2–3 cm, without traction.

The vagus nerves must, systematically, be identified and protected.

*Remark*: The dissection of the hiatus and lower part of the oesophagus into the mediastinum could be often very delicate. The division of the posterior attachments of the cardia on the diaphragm allows to enlarge the retro-oesophageal window. A

**Fig. 3.7** The pleura shall be protected during the intra-mediastinal dissection

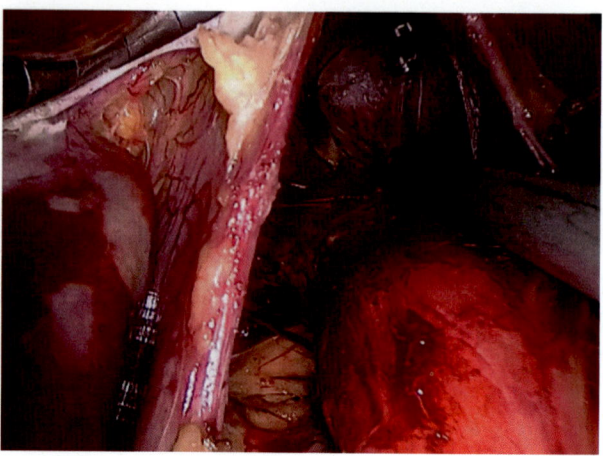

left diaphragmatic artery can be found crossing through that space, in some cases, and this must be kept in mind.

*Risks*: Perforation of the oesophagus, pneumothorax and bleeding if dissection is not careful.

*Prevention:* The rule of "*dissection first of the oesophageal hiatus and not of the oesophagus*" must be respected to avoid any oesophageal perforation. This risk can be minimised by retro-oesophageal dissection in contact with the crura. If there is a large diaphragmatic artery or other unusual vessels, they must be carefully dissected, coagulated or clipped to avoid an undesirable haemorrhage that makes difficult to continue the dissection at this closed and deep area.

Intra-mediastinal dissection shall be done under direct vision, not blindly, preferably with a 30 or 45° optic, and it shall be sufficiently large although not too excessive, in order to avoid negative effects. The pleura shall also be viewed and protected during dissection, to avoid a tear that can lead to a pneumothorax (Fig. 3.7).

### 3.3.1.3 Step-3: Preparation and Mobilisation of the Gastric Fundus

This step involves mobilisation of the gastric fundus, which is used to create the anti-reflux valve. This requires the section of the gastrosplenic ligament and the first short vessels (Fig. 3.8).

*Remark*: The systematic section of the short gastric vessels is to enable the realisation of a tension-free valve (floppy Nissen). Otherwise, if the technique used is the Nissen-Rossetti, it does not require this cutting.

*Recommendation*: This division shall only concern some of the short vessels, not all of the great curvature. Only three or four of the superior short gastric vessels need to be severed; an extensive release of the large curvature of the stomach starting to lower the pole of the spleen is not desirable. The dissection shall continue to the left crus, to liberate the posterior side of the fundus. In certain cases, division of the posterior fundic artery maybe necessary.

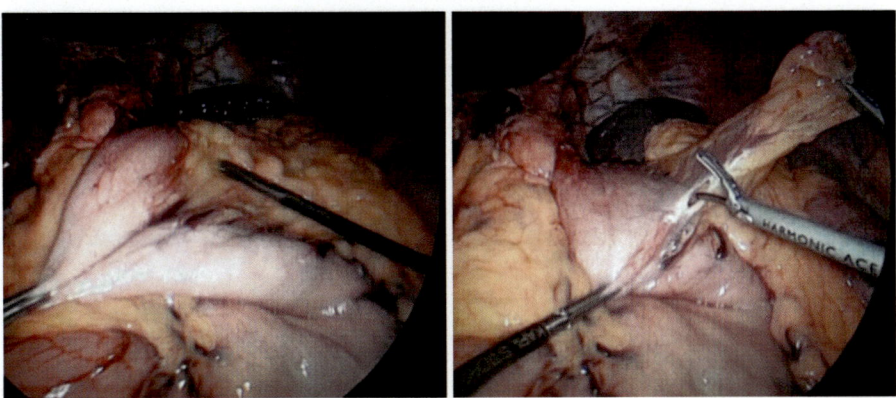

**Fig. 3.8** Section of gastrosplenic ligament with the first short vessels

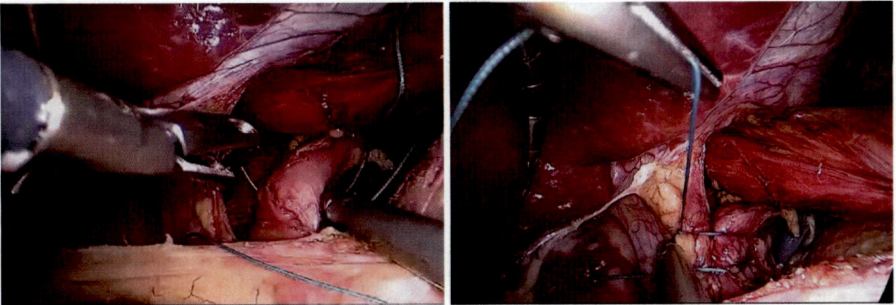

**Fig. 3.9** Approximation of diaphragmatic pillars (cruroplasty)

Monopolar or bipolar cautery, clips, ultrasonic scissors or a vessel sealing device may be used to cut and divide the short gastric vessels.

*Landmarks-1* (Dr. Cadiére) [30]; Dissection of gastrosplenic ligament starts at where the short vessels stop orienting towards the transverse colon (EMC 1995).

*Landmarks-2,* (Dr. Dallemagne) [11]: The ligament is first divided in its cephalad origin where some fat folds may be found (WebSurg), (*J Coeliochir*).

*Risks*: Injury to the spleen, bleeding.

*Prevention*: Dissection of short gastric vessels must be very careful, especially in obese patients. A short gastric vessel poorly controlled may cause local bleeding diffusing into the gastrophrenic ligament and make the following mobilisation difficult. The use of modern haemostatic instruments considerably facilitates a secure haemostasis.

### 3.3.1.4 Step-4. Approximation of Diaphragmatic Pillars (Cruroplasty)

Systematic approximation of the pillars is essential. It not only contributes to restoring one of the elements of the anti-reflux barrier but also stabilises the anti-reflux valve inside the abdominal cavity and prevents the appearance of a para-oesophageal hernia (Fig. 3.9).

**Fig. 3.10** Hiatal repair
with mesh

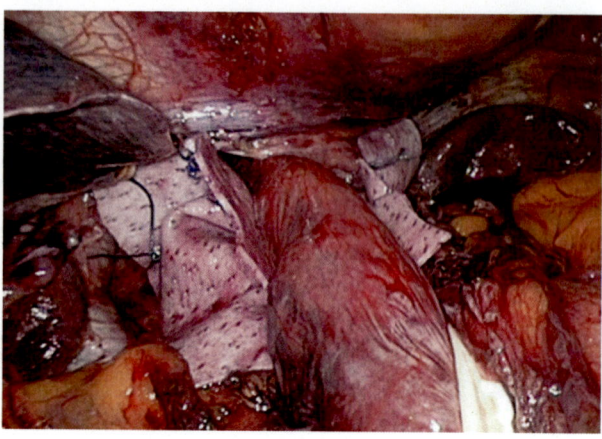

Hiatal repair with mesh reinforcement may reduce hernia recurrence, especially in patients with a large hiatal hernia or in a complex REDO surgery. However, mesh-related complications have to be considered (Fig. 3.10), (Video 3.7).

Video 3.7: Hiatal repair with mesh

*Remarks*: Closure of the crus can be done in front or behind of the oesophagus. Posterior closure seems more anatomical. Anterior closure may be used in cases of very large hiatal defects, but it involves sutures under high tension. In those cases, it is when there may be some interest in the use of mesh reinforcement as a possible solution. However, mesh-related complications have to be considered.

- Indeed, significant and persistent postoperative dysphagia is often due to a too tight closure of the pillars. This may become a valve problem (EMC-3).
- Two or three points of interrupted non-absorbable sutures of 0 or 2/0 are usually sufficient to assure proper repair the hiatal defect posterior to the oesophagus.

*Recommendation:* At the beginning of surgeon's experience, it is recommended to place a 55 French "bougie" into the oesophagus to avoid strangulation, which will result in a dysphagia.
*Risks*:

- Haemorrhage by lesion of the VCI or the aorta
- Laceration of the crus by too tight sutures
- Immediate dysphagia due to a too tight closure of the pillars

*Prevention:* Be careful, by placing the first point inferior; do not touch the aorta when dealing with the left crus or the inferior vena cava when dealing with the right crus (Fig. 3.11).

**Fig. 3.11** Be careful not to hurt the inferior vena cava by loading the right crus

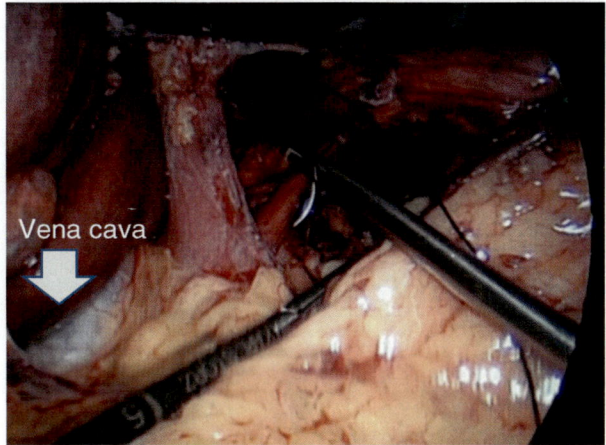

The sutures on the pillars should not be too tight to avoid laceration on the muscle fibres; these can lead to recurrence. Just approaching the crus shall be sufficient and effective.

An instrument of 10 cm—the width of a finger—introduced without difficulty between the oesophagus and the last suture ensures that the closure of the crus is not stenotic.

At the beginning of surgeon's experience, it is recommended to place a 55 French "bougie" into the oesophagus to accurately size the oesophagus and to avoid any strangulation, which will result in dysphagia. But utmost care is necessary to avoid oesophageal perforation!!!

The placement of an oesophageal dilator during the creation of laparoscopic fundoplication is advisable as it leads to decreased postoperative dysphagia but should be weighed against a small risk of oesophageal injury. A 56 French "bougie" has been found effective but the evidence is limited.

### 3.3.1.5 Step-5: Creation of the Fundus Valve (Fundoplication)

The last step of the operation is the creation and fixation of the anti-reflux valve.

The posterior-superior part of the gastric fundus is brought to the right of the oesophagus through the posterior oesophageal window. The two parts of the valve are to be united in the anterior surface of the oesophagus by three non-absorbable sutures (Fig. 3.12).

*Remarks*

- If a proper dissection was done to get a large retro-oesophageal window and adequate mobilisation of the large curvature, this valve will move easily through this retro-oesophageal window and will be maintained without any traction.

*Recommendation*

- Verification of the absence of tension and play in the valve by the "bath towel movement" (go-and-back) in the posterior area.

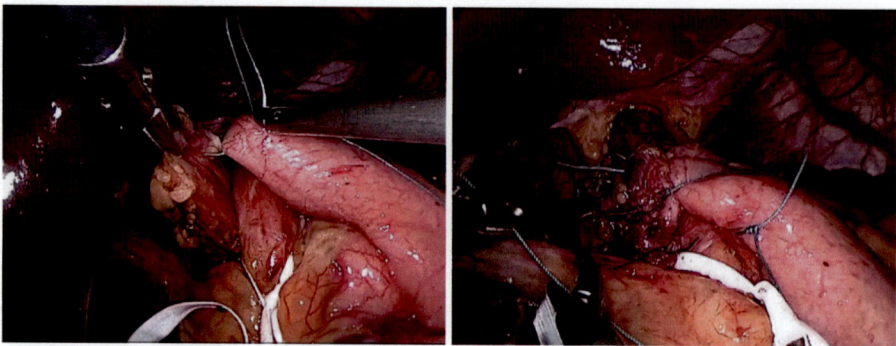

**Fig. 3.12** Creation of the fundus valve (fundoplication)

- The valve should be positioned at the level of the Z line, 1–1.5 cm above the anatomical junction.
- The best length of the valve is about 2 cm in the case of a floppy Nissen.
- It is important to have a good anchorage of the fundoplication on the gastro-oesophageal junction; otherwise it can slip rapidly.
- The placement of an oesophageal dilator during the creation of a laparoscopic fundoplication is advisable as it leads to decreased postoperative dysphagia.
- The valve must be fixed to avoid slipping, usually by two sutures which pass the anterior wall of the oesophagus and at the right of the anterior vagus nerve.

*Risks*: The placement of a 50–60 French "bougie" can be effective but must be balanced with a low risk of oesophageal injury due to lack of care when placing it into the oesophagus.

*Prevention*

- One or two sutures passing the anterior wall of the oesophagus to prevent an eventual slipping into the thorax must fix the valve.
- During this fixation, be careful to avoid taking within the suture the branches of the anterior vagus nerve; this may cause vagal damage.
- The valve can be fixed also to the phreno-oesophageal ligament in order to give good anchorage to the fundoplication.
- When the anaesthetist pushes the dilator in the oesophagus, do not forget to release the tape retractors at the cardia, to avoid a possible perforation of the oesophagus.

## 3.4    Postoperative Complications: Failures

According to Guidelines of SAGES (Society of American Gastrointestinal and Endoscopic Surgeons) [31], there is a failure rate of 10–15 % in spite of a successful outcome in 85–90 % of patients up to 5 years after primary anti-reflux surgery. Failure is usually defined as persistent, recurrent or new-onset symptoms.

The main symptoms of failure are:

- Recurrent reflux symptoms
- Gas-bloat syndrome
- Dysphagia

### 3.4.1 Recurrent Reflux Symptoms

Persistent and recurrent reflux can be due to intrathoracic wrap migration, disruption of the wrap, slipping and/or telescoping. Recurrent reflux symptoms such as heartburn and regurgitation are the main complaints after unsuccessful anti-reflux surgery and are found in 61 % of patients with failure [32].

A variety of symptoms as inability to belch, gastric fullness, early satiety, diarrhoea, nausea and vomiting can occur postoperatively; some due to an overly tight wrap or an overly tight crural repair, others secondary to vagal damage.

### 3.4.2 Gas-Bloat Syndrome

The gas-bloat syndrome corresponds to a series of symptoms attributed to the inability to belch. The main complaint is postprandial bloating. Several factors are evoked to explain this symptomatology as the inability of the oeso-gastric junction to open in response to gastric distension. Some are caused by an overly tight wrap or by an overly tight crural repair. Iatrogenic vagus nerve damage causing gastroparesis can also cause this kind of symptoms.

### 3.4.3 Dysphagia

Troublesome dysphagia is the other most frequent symptom in failed anti-reflux surgery.

Dysphagia for solid food is common in the early postoperative period. This is probably dysphagia caused by the operative oedema, and it disappears spontaneously, often, in two or three months. This is functional rather than mechanical and, as such, does not need surgical correction. It is influenced by the ability of the patient to control his/hers emotions and eating habits.

One of the reasons for functional failure after primary anti-reflux surgery is misdiagnosis. These patients frequently have a primary functional disorder other than GERD such as achalasia, diffuse oesophageal spasm, nutcracker oesophagus, eosinophilic oesophagitis or scleroderma. Another possible cause for failure after primary anti-reflux surgery is that a wrong procedure was used in patients with severe oesophageal dysmotility or motility disorder.

If the intensity of dysphagia does not decrease after the third month and does not disappear, at the sixth month, it must be considered as a mechanical dysphagia, and this requires surgical correction. Accurate diagnosis must be made before any surgery.

Severe dysphagia requires early endoscopic exploration and, whenever appropriate, endoscopic dilation. If symptoms persist, revision surgery has to be envisaged.

The causes of persistent dysphagia can be intrathoracic wrap migration, slipping, telescoping, para-oesophageal herniation, mesh migration, excessive fibrosis (mesh-related or not) and/or an overly tight wrap or overly tight crural repair.

Excessive dysphagia and intractable pain and/or dyspnoea in the early postoperative course require immediate revision after appropriate investigations. In all other failure scenarios, the first-line therapy should be medical and/or supportive.

### 3.4.4 Some Remarks

#### 3.4.4.1 Postoperative "Diaphragmatic Stressors"
One study has suggested that early postoperative gagging, belching and vomiting (especially when associated with gagging) are predisposing factors for anatomical failure and the need for revision [33].

In addition, hiatal hernias >3 cm at original operation have been reported to be predictors for anatomic failure.

#### 3.4.4.2 Psychological Disease and Intervention
One study concluded that a 270° partial fundoplication had better outcomes in patients with major depression compared with a 360° fundoplication due to a lower incidence of postoperative dysphagia and gas-bloat syndrome [34].

#### 3.4.4.3 Oesophageal Function
Patients with nonspecific spastic oesophageal motor disorders (such as nutcracker oesophagus, hypertensive LES syndrome) have been reported to be at increased risk for postoperative heartburn, regurgitation and dysphagia after a 360° wrap [35].

Symptoms should be the primary indication for any redo anti-reflux surgery. All patients seeking treatment for symptomatic failure after anti-reflux surgery should be evaluated to identify possible causes of failure. Investigative techniques include endoscopy, manometry, oesophageal 24-h pH monitoring, barium studies and scintigraphy.

### 3.5  REDO

Redo anti-reflux surgery is required in 3–6 % of all patients who undergo primary anti-reflux surgery and should always begin with a clear definition of the anatomy [1].

Anatomical alterations such as recurrent hernia or a bilobed and twisted stomach have been described as reasons for failure and subsequent redo anti-reflux surgery. However, anatomical disturbance without symptoms should never be the only reason for redo surgery. Symptoms should be the primary indication for redo anti-reflux surgery. Conversely, postoperative anatomy as evaluated by endoscopy and/or barium studies can be normal in patients who still have symptoms.

Anatomical changes after laparoscopic anti-reflux procedures can be classified into several categories, including intrathoracic wrap migration, wrap disruption, telescoping, para-oesophageal herniation, a tight wrap or a tight crural repair and a bilobed or twisted stomach. In the case of any of these conditions, there has to be careful anatomical dissection and proper rearrangement before creating a new fundoplication.

Revisional surgery should be performed by specialised gastrointestinal surgeons with extensive experience in the field, in a high-volume centre. The surgeon's technical armamentarium for revisional surgery should include all laparoscopic, endoscopic and thoracoscopic procedures (Collis), as well as all open procedures, including major resections, if they seem necessary to solve the problem.

## 3.6    Summary

Today, the laparoscopic anti-reflux surgery is the treatment of choice for GERD, and all types of fundoplication can be carried out in good conditions, in accordance with well-defined rules.

Surgical complications of the laparoscopic techniques for GERD are generally rare and due to the non-compliance with well-standardised rules, also lack of experience of the operator. In the beginning, during the initial learning phase, this is one of the main risk factors for complications [13].

Complications of laparoscopic treatment of GERD can be classified as preoperative (minor or serious) and postoperative failures (immediate or delayed).

Intra-operative complications of laparoscopic anti-reflux procedures are essentially traumatic and involve mainly the oesophagus, stomach, pleura and vessels, with consequent haemorrhage, perforations, pneumothorax and some other less frequent.

Haemorrhagic complications are rarely reported in the literature and usually without vital impact (rare cause of conversions and transfusions), whereas perforation of hollow organs as stomach and especially oesophagus can be more important, even catastrophic.

The risk of oesophageal perforation can be minimised by the retro-oesophageal dissection remaining in contact with the pillars of the diaphragm. To avoid perforation, we must not forget the basic principles of "Dissection at start of the oesophageal hiatus and not of oesophagus".

The consequences vary as detection is early or late. If it is discovered during surgery, there is a good chance to repair, perhaps laparoscopically, with good recovery. Otherwise, with unnoticed oesophageal perforation, all of it can lead to a very severe complication, even death.

Gastric perforations are rarer than oesophageal, while pneumothorax and the pneumomediastinum are in fact very frequent and less serious complications.

Postoperative complications depend on a good diagnostic, choice of an adequate technique, experience and skills of the surgeon and the general condition of each case. The main symptoms of failure are recurrent reflux, gas-bloat syndrome and dysphagia.

Heartburn and regurgitation are the main complaints after unsuccessful anti-reflux surgery and are found in the majority of patients with unsuccessful result. Persistent and recurrent reflux can be due to intrathoracic wrap migration, disruption of the wrap, slipping and/or telescoping.

The gas-bloat syndrome corresponds to a series of symptoms attributed to the inability to belch. Some can be due to an overly tight wrap or an overly tight crural repair, others secondary to iatrogenic vagal damage.

Troublesome dysphagia is the other most frequent symptom in failed anti-reflux surgery. Dysphagia for solid food is common in early postoperative period. This is probably the dysphagia consequence of operative oedema as it disappears often spontaneously in 2 or 3 months. If the degree of dysphagia does not decrease after the third month and does not disappear by the sixth month, it must be considered as a mechanical dysphagia that requires surgical correction. This may be after some trial of endoscopic dilation.

## References

1. Fuchs KH, Babic B, Dallemagne B, Fingerhut A, Furnee E, Granderath F, Horvath P, Kardos P, Pointner R, Savarino E, Van Herwaarden-Lindeboom M, Zaninotto G (2014) European Association of Endoscopic Surgery (EAES), EAES recommendations for the management gastroesophageal reflux disease. Surg Endosc 28(6):1753–1773
2. Nissen R (1956) Eine einfache operation zur Beeinflussung des Refluxo¨sophagitis. Schweiz Med Wschr 86:590–592
3. Toupet A (1963) Technique de oesophagogastroplastie appliquée à la cure radicale des hernies hiatales et comme complément de l'operation Heller dans les cardiospasmes. Mem Acd Chir 89:384–389
4. Katkhouda N, Khalil N, Manhas S, Grant S, Velmahos GC, Umbach TW, Kaiser AM (2002) André Toupet: surgeon technician par excellence. Ann Surg 235:591–599
5. Belsey R (1977) Mark IV repair of hiatal hernia by the transthoracic approach. World J Surg 1:475–483
6. Hill LD (1967) An effective operation for hiatal hernia and eight years appraisal. Ann Surg 166:681–692
7. Rosseti M, Hell K (1977) Fundoplication for the treatment of gastroesophageal reflux in hiatal hernia. World J Surg 1:439–444
8. DeMeester TR, Bonavina L, Albertucci M (1986) Nissen fundoplication or gastroesophageal reflux disease. Evaluation of primary repair in 100 consecutive patients. Ann Surg 204(1):9–20
9. Dallemagne B, Weerts JM, Jehaes C, Markiewicz S, Lombard R (1991) Laparoscopic Nissen fundoplication: preliminary report. Surg Laparos Endosc 1:138–143
10. Dallemagne B, Weerts JM, Markiewicz S, Devandre JM, Wahlen C, Monami B, JEHAES C (2006) Clinical results of laparoscopic fundoplication ten years after surgery. Surg Endosc 20:159–165
11. Dallemagne B (2013) Comment je réalise une "floppy" fundoplication de Nissen. J Coeliochirurgie 85:35–41
12. Di Martino N, Brillantino A, Torelli F, Marano L (2010) What's new in the laparoscopic surgical treatment of GERD. What' is new in Laparoscopic surgery? Edizioni Minerva Medica 2:7–13
13. Rantanen TK, Oksala NK, Oksala AK, Salo JA, Sihvo EI (2008) Complications in antireflux surgery: national-based analysis of laparoscopic and open fundoplications. Arch Surg 143(4):359–365
14. Watson DI, Bajgrie RJ, Jamieson GG (1996) A learning curve for laparoscopic fundoplication-definable, avoidable or waste of time? Ann Surg 224:198–203

15. Champault G (1994) Traitement par laparoscopie: 940 cas expérience français. Ann Chir 48:159–164
16. Dallemagne B, Taziaux P, Weerts JM, Jehaes C, Markiewicz S (1995) Chiryrgie laparoscopique du gastro-oesphagien. Ann Chir 49:30–36
17. Niebisch S, Fleming FJ, Galey KM, Wilshire CL, Jones CE, Little VR et al (2012) Perioperative risk of laparoscopic fundoplication: safer than previously reported-analysis of the American College of Surgeons. National Surgical Quality Improvement Program 2005 to 2009. J Am Coll Surg 215:61–68
18. Sodji M, Durand-Fontanier S, Pech de Laclause B, Valleix D, Segol P, Descottes B (1999) Complications des cures laparoscopiques du reflux gastro-oesphagien. In: Descottes B, Samama G, Segol P (eds) Complications De La Chirurgie Abdominale Sous Video-Laparoscopie. Rapport présenté au 101. Cngres Français de Chirurgie, Arnette-Paris
19. Hinder RA, Perdikis G, Klinger PJ, Devault-Kenneth R (1997) The surgical option for gastro-esophageal disease. Am J Med 103:144–148
20. Watson DI, Gourlay R, Globe J, Reed MWR, Johnson AG, Stoddard CJ (1994) Prospective randomised trial of laparoscopic (LNF) versus open (ONF) Nissen fundoplication. Gut 35(Supp 2):S15, Abst W58
21. Gotler DC, Smithers BM, Rhodes M, Menzies B, Branicky FJ, Nathanson L (1996) Laparoscopic Nissen fundoplication 200 consecutive cases. Gut 18:487–491
22. Collet D, Zerbib F, Ledaguenel P, Perissat J (1998) Fundoplicature pour reflux gastro-oesphagien. Ann Chir 51(10):1084–1091
23. Joris JL, Chichr J, Lamy ML (1995) Pneumothorax during laparoscopic fundoplication: diagnosis and treatment with positive end-expiratory pressure. Anesth Analg 81:993–1000
24. SWIDE C, Nyberg PF (1996) Cardiac trauma; an unusual cause of dysrhythmias and electrocardiographic changes during laparoscopic Nissen fundoplication. Anesthesiology 85:209–211
25. Boccara G, Lopez S, Huguet M, Mann C, Colson P (1998) Myopéricardite aigue dans les suites d'une cure laparoscopique de reflux gastro-oesphagienne. Ann Fr Anesth Reanim 17:1148–1151
26. Farlo J, Thawgathurari D, Michil M, Yaker K, Sullivan E, Morgan E (1998) Cardiac tamponade during laparoscopic Nissen fundoplication. Eur J Anesthesiol 5:246–247
27. Peters JH, Heimbucher J, Kauer WK, Incarbone R, Bremner CG, Demeester TR (1995) Clinical and physiologic comparison of laparoscopic and open Nissen fundoplication. J Am Coll Surg 180:385–392
28. Eyuboglu E, Ipek T (2011) Laparoscopic floppy Nissen fundoplication: 16 years of experience from the historical clinic of Rudolph Nissen. Hepatogastroenterology 58(110–111):1607–1610. doi:10.5754/hge10654. Epub 2011 Jul 15
29. Ipek T, Eyuboglu E, Ozmen V (2010) Partial splenic infarction as a complication of laparoscopic floppy nissen fundoplication. J Laparoendosc Adv Surg Tech A 20(4):333–337. doi:10.1089/lap.2009.0409
30. Cadière GB (1995) Traitement du reflux gastro-oesphagien par coelioscopie. Encyclopèdie Médco-Chirurgicale: EMC 40(189):1–10
31. SAGES Guidelines Committee; Stefanidis D, Hope WW, Kohn GP, Reardon PR, Richardson WS, Fanelli RD (2010) Guidelines for surgical treatment of gastroesophageal reflux disease (GERD). SAGES – Society of American Gastrointestinal and Endoscopic Surgeons. Surg Endosc 24(11):2647–2669. http://www.sages.org
32. Furnè EJ, Draaisma WA, Broeders IA, Smout AJ, Vlek AL, Gooszen GG (2008) Predictors of symptomatic and objective outcomes after surgical reintervention for failed antireflux surgery. Br J Surg 95:1369–1374
33. Iqbal A, Kakarlapudi GV, Awad ZT, Haynatzki G, Turaga KK, Karu A, Fritz K, Haider M, Mittal SK, Filipi CJ (2006) Assessment of diaphragmatic stressors as risk factors for symptomatic failure of laparoscopic Nissen fundoplication. J Gastrointest Surg 10:12–21
34. Kamolz T, Granderath FA, Pointner R (2003) Does major depression in patients with gastroesophageal reflux disease affect the outcome of laparoscopic antireflux surgery. Surg Endosc 17:55–60
35. Winslow ER, Clouse RE, Desai KM, Frisella P, Gunsberger T, Soper NJ, Klingensmith ME (2003) Influence of spastic motor disorders of the esophageal body on outcome from laparoscopic antireflux surgery. Surg Endosc 17:738–745

# Complications, Reoperations, Tips and Tricks in Laparoscopic Colorectal Surgery

**4**

T.A. Rockall and D. Singh-Ranger

## 4.1 Introduction

Laparoscopic surgery for colorectal disease demands advanced laparoscopic skills and has the potential for serious complications both intraoperatively and in the post-operative phase. Some are specific to the laparoscopic approach; others are equally common with both laparoscopic and open approaches, but methods to deal with these complications in the laparoscopic environment are often more challenging and require knowledge of specific techniques in order to avoid conversion to open surgery.

## 4.2 Intraoperative Complications

### 4.2.1 Haemorrhage

Intraoperative haemorrhage can occur in a number of different scenarios, and specific problems related to colorectal surgery are discussed. Port-site haemorrhage, for example, will not be dealt with here.

Arterial haemorrhage from a major colorectal artery is immediately evident and occurs as a result of inadvertent division (partial or complete) during the dissection of a vascular pedicle. Inappropriate or improper use of an energy device can also lead to poor sealing of major vessels which might result in either immediate or delayed haemorrhage. Vessels may also be avulsed due to inappropriate traction

Electronic supplementary material The online version of this chapter (doi:10.1007/978-3-319-19623-7_4) contains supplementary material, which is available to authorized users.

T.A. Rockall, MD, FRCS (✉) • D. Singh-Ranger, MS, FRCS
Minimal Access Therapy Training Unit, Royal Surrey County Hospital NHS Trust, Guildford, UK
e-mail: tim.rockall@btinternet.com

although this more commonly leads to venous haemorrhage. Blood loss from this kind or injury can be rapid and requires prompt action to firstly control the blood loss and secondly to secure the vessel.

Control of haemorrhage can often be achieved with the application of an appropriate grasper to the vessel if it is visible and if there is sufficient length of vessel for a grasper to be applied. Circumstances in which there is no cuff of vessel—for example, where the inferior mesenteric artery (IMA) has been divided flush with the aorta—are more difficult. Where a grasping instrument or the energy device cannot be judiciously applied, then immediate application of pressure with a small swab accurately over the source will usually control the bleeding. Once the active blood loss is controlled, there is time to contemplate how best to proceed. Appropriate instrumentation can be made available such as a clip applicator, suction irrigation and sutures and importantly extra ports deployed in order to utilise assistance for application of pressure or suction irrigation. In any circumstance where blood loss is not rapidly controlled, then immediate conversion to open access is indicated.

When there is a cuff of a divided vessel visible, then application of a suitable sized clip is often the best method of control. There is however no place for blind clip application, and this needs to be done in a controlled fashion. If the energy source can be safely applied to a vessel of appropriate size for the device, then this is also acceptable method of control. The device should completely control the haemorrhage when applied before activation of the energy source.

Avulsion injuries are the result of poor surgical technique and can be difficult to control as the proximal end of the vessel may not be visible. It may be possible to control the bleeding with pressure before proceeding as above; but if the bleeding source cannot be found, conversion to open surgery is recommended for uncontrolled haemorrhage. More minor bleeding that is controlled with pressure may be manageable by prolonging the application of pressure and incorporating haemostatic materials.

Energy devices need to be used as per the manufacturer's recommendations. If used incorrectly or on inappropriately sized vessels, the haemorrhage can result either immediately or in a delayed fashion. Ultrasonic devices (e.g. Harmonic ACE™ (Ethicon Endosurgery)), intelligent bipolar vessel-sealing device (e.g. LigaSure™, Covidien) and hybrid energy sources (e.g. Thunderbeat™, Olympus), are the most widely used devices. The standard Harmonic ACE is licensed to divide and seal vessels not more than 5 mm and the newer Harmonic ACE 7 up to 7 mm. LigaSure and Thunderbeat also seal vessels up to 7 mm. Division of larger vessels with these devices alone is not recommended, and in all cases, consideration needs to be given to vessel characteristics (e.g. calcification) and to using the correct technique and power settings. In all cases, vascular pedicles should not be divided flush with the major proximal blood vessel (i.e. the aorta when dividing the IMA). Haemorrhage is both more likely and much more difficult to control. A pedicle of at least 1 cm is advisable. Vessels should be dissected and clearly identified prior to division as this allows the visualisation of the true vessel diameter and permits separate division of artery and vein. If this proves difficult, then a vascular stapling device is a good alternative (use of the correct white stapling cartridge for vascular division is necessary). For bipolar sealing devices, it is imperative that the vessel should only be divided once the instrument has indicated that the seal is complete. This is automatically detected by simultaneous measurement of the impedance of the tissue as it desiccates and seals. Ultrasonic technology is different in that the device cuts and seals simultaneously. For the seal on a major vessel to be effective, tension on the pedicle must be diminished and the "minimum" indicator set to the lowest possible (Setting one on the Harmonic ACE) to maximise coagulation and seal. Activation should be with the instrument fully closed and with no pressure on the active blade. Diseased vessels, especially those that are heavily calcified, may not seal well and clips should be applied.

Haemorrhage from a staple line is not uncommon even where the correct vascular (white) cartridge has been used. It is usually minor and stops spontaneously. If arterial and spurting, then judicious application of a clip is effective. If just oozing, then this can be effectively controlled with a swab and the bleeding will stop spontaneously.

Anatomical variation of vasculature is important principally for the understanding of the development of ischaemia and where appropriate colonic division should take place. The ileocolic artery has the most constant position originating independently from the right side of the superior mesenteric artery (SMA) in 63 % of individuals. In the remainder, it forms a common trunk with the right colic artery. The right colic and middle colic arteries can be absent, and knowledge of this is crucial when deciding upon the amount of right colon to transect. The right colic artery has the greatest variation amongst individuals. In 40 % it originates as a separate branch from the SMA and in 30 % from the middle colic artery and in 20 % is absent. In such a situation, the right colon will receive its vascular supply from the ascending and descending branches of the ileocolic and right branch of the middle colic arteries (Fig. 4.1). With this scenario, a mid ascending colon neoplasm would require division of the ileocolic and right branch of middle colic vessels. Likewise, for a caecal or proximal ascending colon neoplasm, dividing the ileocolic vessels at their origin may result in excision of a greater length of colon as the right colic vessels may be part of the common trunk. If possible, the courses of these vessels should be noted prior to division.

Alternatively, as division of the appropriate vessel is crucial, extracorporeal division may be preferable once the colon has been mobilised, if the anatomy is uncertain.

The middle colic artery usually originates from the SMA at the inferior border of the uncinate process of the pancreas. In 25 % it can be absent and in 10 % there may be an accessory or double vessel. The right and left branches of this artery arise at the middle of the transverse colon. If intracorporeal division of the right branch is contemplated, then search for it should begin from the middle of the transverse colon.

The inferior mesenteric artery (IMA) provides the blood supply to the descending and sigmoid colons and upper rectum. It originates from the anterior surface of the abdominal aorta although its position is not constant, lying anywhere along a line from the origin of the SMA to the aortic bifurcation. In most cases, the origin is

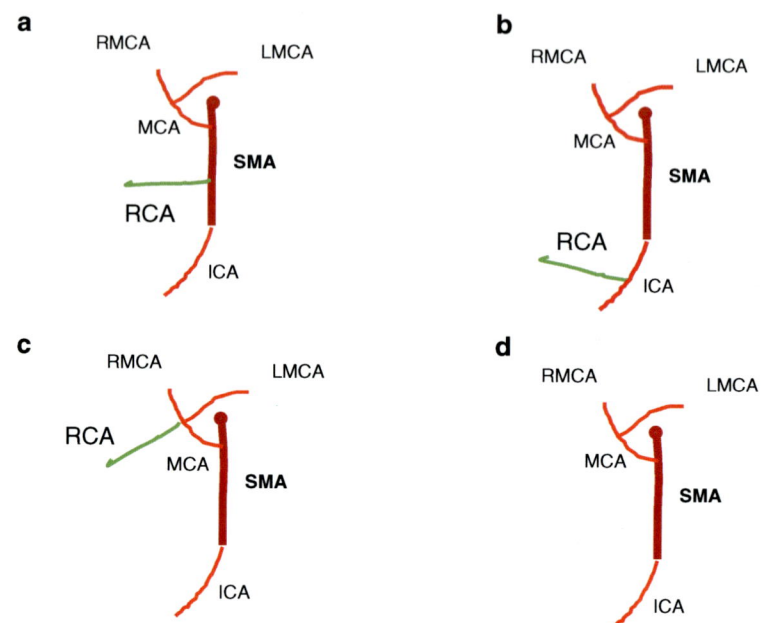

**Fig. 4.1** Division of relevant pedicles in relation to tumour location in the right colon. (**a**) Right colic artery arising from the superior mesenteric artery. (**b**) Right colic artery arising from the ileocolic trunk. (**c**) Right colic artery arising from the middle colic artery. (**d**) Right colic artery absent. *SMA* superior mesenteric artery, *RCA* right colic artery, *MCA* middle colic artery, *RMCA* right branch of middle colic artery, *LMCA* left branch of middle colic artery

just below or under the third part of the duodenum. From here the artery runs obliquely and crosses the pelvic brim at the aortic bifurcation. To prevent early injury, the first incision used to commence medial to lateral dissection should be made at the root of the sigmoid mesentery anterior to the right common iliac artery, rather than over the sacral promontory. The left ureter and gonadal vessels pass close to the IMA origin. They must be recognised and dissected clear (if necessary) before the IMA is divided. The diameter of the IMA is 50 % that of the SMA. The principles that apply to division of arterial vessels with modern energy sources and stapling devices are equally relevant to this vessel. Rarely does the IMA have to be divided at its origin. The left colic artery provides a significant blood supply to the splenic flexure. It is important to know the anatomical variations of the LCA as if this is inadvertently divided; there is a risk that this section of the colon will become ischaemic necessitating splenic flexure mobilisation and more proximal division of colon. In over 50 % of individuals, the LCA arises as a separate branch of the IMA, and in the remainder it forms a common trunk with the first sigmoidal artery (Fig. 4.2). A useful tip in identifying the LCA is to locate the IMV as the former usually travels adjacent to the latter.

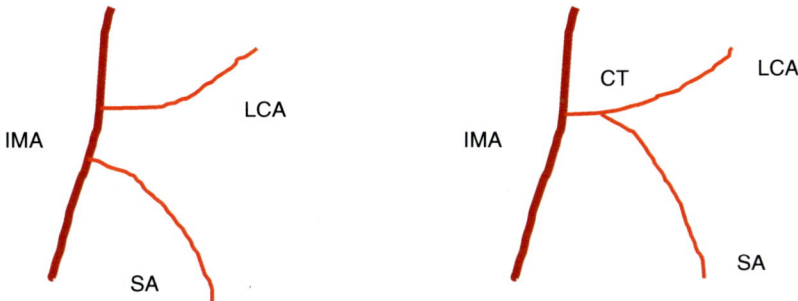

**Fig. 4.2** Anatomical variation of left colic artery. *IMA* inferior mesenteric artery, *LCA* left colic artery, *SA* sigmoidal artery, *CT* common trunk

### 4.2.1.1 Other Vascular Injuries

Injury to the common iliac arteries and external and internal iliac veins is possible, either as a trocar injury or during medial to lateral mobilisation of the left colon and total mesorectal excision of the rectum (TME). Blood loss can be significant and this can have an impact on anastomotic integrity (see below). Repair can be achieved laparoscopically, but conversion to an open procedure and specialist vascular intervention is desirable for patient safety.

### 4.2.2   Ischaemia

Ischaemia of either the proximal or distal parts of an anastomosis will usually result in anastomotic dehiscence. Ischaemia insufficient to cause necrosis may later present with stricture but this is unusual. With a standardised approach to segmental colorectal resection, ischaemia is unusual but may result when there is anatomical variation of the colonic vasculature as previously discussed or probably most commonly during left-sided resection when insufficient mobilisation of the splenic flexure causes the surgeon to divide the left colon too distally in an ischaemic segment. This is most likely in cases with poor marginal artery perfusion. Mostly ischaemia of the proximal conduit can be avoided by fully mobilising the splenic flexure when necessary so that a tension-free anastomosis can be constructed using a well-vascularised bowel. Mostly ischaemia is evident from the colour of the bowel when exteriorised. There may even be a clear demarcation. A tip to ensure that the bowel is well vascularised is to always divide the marginal vessel extracorporeally. Once the level of planned division is identified, the marginal artery is divided between clips. The distal end is tied and the proximal end then gently released to observe arterial blood flow. If there is no active bleeding, then a more proximal site should be chosen. When the bowel itself is divided, there should be bright red mucosal bleeding. There may be a role for the use of Indocyanine Green (ICG) fluorescence to assess perfusion if the technology is available.

Increased blood flow to the colorectal or colo-anal anastomosis may be achieved in the following ways.

1. A more proximal division of the left colon following full mobilisation of the splenic flexure.
2. Preserve the ascending left colic artery where possible.
3. Create a side to end anastomosis.

When balancing the requirement to mobilise the splenic flexure to obtain length with preserving the ascending left colic artery, it is often feasible to divide the inferior mesenteric vein high at the lower border of the pancreas but leave the ascending colic artery intact.

## 4.2.3   Organ Injury

This section discusses the organs and structures most likely to be injured during a laparoscopic colorectal resection. It includes a discussion on splenic, pancreatic and gastric injury during splenic flexure mobilisation, ureteric injury during left-sided resections and total mesorectal excision and bladder trauma.

### 4.2.3.1 Spleen, Pancreas and Stomach

Splenic flexure mobilisation is often necessary for anterior resection of the rectum or even for more proximal segmental resection. The aim being to achieve a tension-free and well-vascularised anastomosis of healthy bowel. To assess adequate length, the planned point of colonic division can be brought down to the transected rectum intracorporeally prior to exteriorisation. Extracorporeally the end of the colonic conduit should reach well past the symphysis pubis following resection of the pathological segment in order to reach the pelvic floor comfortably when replaced intracorporeally for anastomosis.

Splenic injury seems to be much less common during laparoscopic surgery than in open surgery. This is because most splenic injuries are a result of traction of the colon, which avulses splenic capsule tissue at the site of congenital adhesion. At open surgery, too much traction can be created and the sites of adhesion are not well seen. Nevertheless, the same problem can occur at laparoscopic surgery, or direct trauma can occur in inexperienced surgeons especially in fat patients with fatty omentum obscuring the natural planes between spleen, omentum and transverse colon. The operator should be aware of potential injury to the spleen, short gastric vessels and pancreas. Excessive colonic retraction can cause bleeding from a tear in the splenic capsule. It can go unrecognised and so should be investigated when blood is noticed pooling in the left upper quadrant. The most likely site for a tear is at the inferior border or hilum. Primary suture repair and/or application of modern haemostatic agents such as fibrin glue or cellular polymer and radiofrequency ablation with pressure should be considered before contemplating a splenectomy [1]. Very effective haemostatic materials are available which are effective even in significant splenic injury, and all abdominal surgeons should be trained in the correct use of these materials. Inappropriate traction on the stomach may result in trauma to the short gastric vessels. During splenic flexure mobilisation, the stomach does not need to be retracted and so should be avoided. There may be times when the lesser sac needs to be entered between the transverse mesocolon and body of pancreas. If this is attempted, strict adherence to the surgical plane between the transverse mesocolon and pancreas is advised. Noting the slight subtle colour difference between pancreatic fat and that of the mesocolon should help guide the dissection.

### 4.2.3.2 The Ureter and Gonadal Vessels

An understanding of embryology is the key to ensuring that injury to the ureter and gonadal vessels is avoided. During development the abdominal musculature encloses the peritoneal "balloon". Situated behind the balloon are the pancreas, kidneys, adrenal glands, the great vessels and abdominal musculature (e.g. psoas, quadratus lumborum). The gastrointestinal bud enters the abdominal cavity at the neck of the balloon and takes with it a lining of peritoneum—the visceral peritoneum. It exits at the pelvic brim and continues on at the mid rectum. Within the abdominal cavity, ascending, descending and sigmoid colonic visceral peritoneum is very closely apposed to the posterior parietal peritoneum. During medial to lateral dissection, these two layers can be separated, and by staying in the correct plane, the ureter and gonadal vessels remain behind the posterior parietal peritoneum. The ureter can be identified by its vermiculation.

The left ureter can be juxtaposed to the origin of the IMA and may be retracted upwards when lifting this vessel. Consequently before dividing the IMA, it is vital to ensure that the ureter is clearly separated.

Ureteric trauma is possible during pelvic dissection for a ventral rectopexy, deep infiltrating endometriosis or rectal resection. There are slight anatomical variations in the course of the pelvic part of the ureter between males and females. Appreciation of these differences helps towards protecting the ureters. After crossing the pelvic brim at the origin of the external iliac artery, the ureters travel along the pelvic sidewall anterior to the internal iliac vessels. At the ischial spine, they turn medially and enter the bladder base above the pelvic floor. In the male, the ureters are crossed by the ductus deferens. During low rectal mobilisation, keeping the dissection below the seminal vesicles will avoid ureteric injury, as it is at this point that they enter the bladder base. In the female, the ureters are "hidden" beneath the broad ligament and then lie on the surface of the lateral cervical ligaments before entering the bladder base in front of the vaginal fornix. Unfamiliarity of their course can result in ureteric division or obstruction by applying a haemostatic clip for bleeding, for example. Stenting of the ureter can be useful to help identify its course and also protect it against injury. However, this procedure is for the most part unnecessary except in a few key situations.

Stage IV endometriosis
Surgery for local recurrence of cancer

Some cases of benign inflammatory disease
Preoperative ureteric dilatation or obstruction
Known congenital renal abnormality
Single kidney

A recognised ureteric transection may be repaired laparoscopically with sutures if the proximal and distal ends can be united without tension (Video 4.1). This is possible where there has been no or minimal tissue loss and there has been no devascularisation of the ureter and where the site of transection is proximal to the bladder. The stent should remain for at least 6 weeks post repair. If a tension-free primary repair is impossible, then reimplantation using a Boari flap may be necessary, and expert help should be sought.

### 4.2.3.3 Bladder

Bladder injury is uncommon as it is directly visualised during laparoscopic dissection. Trauma may occur when a port trocar is passed through the bladder. Decompressing the bladder by catheterisation should prevent this and also improves the view of the pelvis and facilitates access and is mandatory for all pelvic surgery. A chronically obstructed bladder is particularly at risk during trocar placement, and care should be taken when inserting suprapubic trocars under direct vision. The bladder is also at risk when making a low transverse suprapubic incision as for specimen extraction during left-sided resection. In all cases, recognition of the injury is the key to avoiding subsequent complications. Injuries to the dome of the bladder should be sutured directly with absorbable sutures making sure the knots are external to the bladder. Integrity of the repair can be tested by filling the bladder via the catheter with sterile water (there is no need to use methylene blue dye). A complex repair benefits from a period of bladder decompression postoperatively. Bladder integrity can be checked by cystography prior to removal of the catheter.

Injuries to the base of the bladder should be very rare. Complex stage IV endometriosis can involve the trigone or bladder wall close to the ureteric orifices. In these cases, specialist urological input is required and preoperative stenting is crucial in allowing a safe bladder repair.

---

## 4.3     Postoperative Complications

### 4.3.1   Anastomotic Leak

Morbidity and mortality following a colorectal anastomotic dehiscence is substantial. A leak following a laparoscopic TME for neoplasia will result in a suboptimal long-term oncological outcome [2]. Restoration of intestinal continuity may not be possible and the patient may be left with a permanent stoma. All steps should be taken to minimise the chances of anastomotic failure, but there will be times that the anastomosis will leak despite adhering to all principles for good anastomotic technique. In situations where a leak is suspected, diagnosis and treatment must be prompt and consideration given to saving the life of the patient and reducing the impact of systemic sepsis as well as potentially "saving the anastomosis" in some situations. Treatment comprises patient support and surgical attention to the leak. This may vary from complete disconnection and an end stoma or primary repair with a defunctioning loop stoma.

### 4.3.1.1 Identification of Risk Factors

In the preoperative phase, it is vital to identify risk factors that increase the risk for an anastomotic leak (Table 4.1). Male sex, comorbidity (including diabetes), a smoking history, long-term and perioperative steroids, high body mass index and preoperative chemoradiotherapy have been shown to be significant for anastomotic leak [3, 4]. Intraoperative factors include faecal contamination, blood loss of 100 ml or more, multiple firings of the staple gun, a level of anastomosis less than 4 cm and operation time of more than 120 min [5, 6]. Intraoperative episodes of hypotension and should be avoided. In 285 patients undergoing elective left-sided resections, severe hypotension (>40 % from baseline) was a significant factor for anastomotic leak [7]. In 223 patients who had a gastrointestinal anastomosis, dehiscence was three times more likely if a vasopressor had been used for pressure support [8]. Supplemental oxygenation in the intra- and postoperative period for 6 h will have a beneficial effect. In a randomised controlled trial of 80 % oxygen during and 6 h after surgery, the risk of leak decreased by 46 % when compared to those having 30 % oxygen [9]. The role of maintaining normothermia in preventing surgical site infections is established. One study has implied that a higher intraoperative temperature predisposed to anastomotic leak and increased length of hospital stay. However, a type I error may well have occurred as the sample size was small ($n = 76$) as were the number of leaks [10].

### 4.3.1.2 Preventive Factors

The bowel ends should be well vascularised and the anastomosis free of tension. Division of the IMA at the origin (high ligation) was thought to be oncologically optimal; however, there is no concrete evidence to suggest a survival advantage with high ligation, although the number of lymph nodes retrieved is better [11]. An

**Table 4.1** Risk factors that increase the risk for anastomotic leak

| Preoperative | Intraoperative |
|---|---|
| Male gender | Low rectal anastomosis (<4 cm) |
| Obesity | Blood loss >100 ml |
| Smoking history | Operation time >120 min |
| Diverticulitis | Multiple staple firings |
| Steroid therapy (long-term and preoperative pulmonary) | End—end stapled colorectal anastomosis |
| | Faecal contamination |
| Preoperative chemoradiotherapy | Intraoperative hypotension |
| | Vasopressor use |
| | Oxygen therapy |

analysis of colonic length revealed an insignificant gain from high vs. low ligation (2.9 ± 1.2 cm vs. 3.1 ± 1.8 cm [p = 0.83]). When combined with a high division of the inferior mesenteric vein (IMV), the length increase was significantly greater (19.1 ± 3.8 vs. 8.8 ± 2.9 cm, p = 0.00089) [12]. A high ligation should be considered if a tension-free anastomosis is not attainable with low ligation and division of the IMV or if preoperative radiology suggests more proximal lymph node metastases. If a tension-free anastomosis is not possible even after division of the inferior mesenteric vein, the splenic flexure should be fully mobilised.

Multiple staple firings to transect the mid to low rectum may increase the risk for anastomotic leak. Most rectal transections can be achieved with one or two firings of a 45- or 60-mm stapler if sufficient mobilisation has been undertaken and all the mesorectum divided. Use of a flexible stapling device and introducing the stapler through a suprapubic port can help achieve good transection even in a narrow pelvis.

Orientation of the proximal colon before fashioning the anastomosis is vital in preventing torsion. Ischaemia of the torted segment can occur with subsequent anastomotic dehiscence. To prevent torsion, it is important to ensure that the taeniae coli follow a straight course, usually along the superomedial surface of the left colon (Video 4.2). Once the colorectal anastomosis has been fashioned, tension-relieving sutures across the anastomosis may be helpful in minimising anastomotic leak. There is evidence to show a fivefold reduction in clinical leak with the technique [13] (Video 4.3). It is also feasible that the anastomosis becomes ischaemic once it has been fashioned. If during laparoscopy the anastomosis is dusky, it is better to redo the anastomosis. The vascularity of bowel on either side of the anastomosis can also be judged for adequacy by intraoperative rigid sigmoidoscopy or colonoscopy. If there is any doubt, then the anastomosis should be refashioned.

### 4.3.1.3 Diagnosis of Anastomotic Leak

An anastomotic leak should be suspected when the patient exhibits signs of the systemic inflammatory response syndrome (SIRS) on postoperative day 3/4. Other subtle signs include a drop in oxygen saturation, rising respiratory rate, a cardiac arrhythmia, neurological complications such as delirium and worsening abdominal pain and/or distension. The suspicion of a leak must be high with a paralytic ileus that fails to resolve after electrolyte and fluid abnormalities have been corrected. Some have suggested that plasma C-reactive protein (CRP) above 140 mg·l$^{-1}$ (on postoperative day 3) is a sensitive and specific surrogate marker for anastomotic leak [14]. Imaging in the form of computerised tomography or Gastrografin enemas are useful, but their interpretation is limited and should be within the context of the clinical signs and symptoms. Early recourse to diagnostic laparoscopy if the suspicion for anastomotic leak is high, irrespective of the findings on radiological imaging. A leak detected early may allow the anastomosis to be preserved and so the threshold for diagnostic laparoscopy should be low. In one systematic review, the sensitivity of computerised tomography (CT) was 68 % [15].

#### 4.3.1.4 Preservation of Anastomosis

There are many ways to attempt to preserve the rectal anastomosis following a leak, but this should not be attempted at the expense of the patient's overall wellbeing. If the colonic conduit is not ischaemic or necrotic, then an attempt at salvaging the anastomosis is potentially worthwhile. For a low rectal anastomosis, access to a posterior leak via the abdomen may be extremely difficult. One method where access to the leak is facilitated is the transanal approach. Transanal endoscopic microsurgery will allow the anastomosis to be clearly seen and permit suture repair (Video 4.4). Alternatively success has been described with the use of specialised vacuum dressing placed in the leak cavity in conjunction with a defunctioning stoma. Laparoscopy can be employed to deal with intra-abdominal contamination.

#### 4.3.1.5 Postoperative Intestinal Obstruction

A sizeable mesenteric window can occur when the anastomosis has been fashioned. Small bowel loops can pass through the window causing mechanical obstruction. It is an infrequent complication but always requires reoperation to rectify. There is no evidence that closing these defects prevents these rare occurrences. The most common event of this type usually follows a left hemicolectomy where the splenic flexure has been excised and a colo-colonic anastomosis fashioned. This leaves a large mesenteric defect into which the small bowel is prone to herniate. The patients are acutely unwell with small bowel obstruction, and cross-sectional imaging will show dilated small bowel in the left side of the abdomen and the left colon/anastomosis pushed to the right. It is usually also associated with signs of anastomotic leak. Preventive methods include retraction of small bowel from the window with interposition of omentum, if possible. Other means by which obstruction may occur is when small bowel rotates around the proximal limb of a defunctioning loop ileostomy. Suture fixation of the small bowel is of little value as a preventive measure and so is not recommended. Repeat laparoscopy should be considered if postoperative mechanical obstruction is suspected within the first few postoperative days.

---

#### Conclusions

Laparoscopic colorectal complications are infrequent but when they occur are potentially serious. The majority of complications are injuries to viscera, organs and vessels with the most significant postoperative one being anastomotic leak from a low rectal anastomosis. Several reasons are responsible for laparoscopic injuries and include the abdominal "blind spot", ineffective retraction of small bowel, poor technique and insufficient knowledge of anatomy and anatomical variations. Unfamiliarity with instrumentation especially energy sources significantly contribute to intraoperative injuries. Division of vascular pedicles should take into account the vessel diameter, limitations of energy source used and the need for adjuncts such as clips and stapling devices. If major haemorrhage from a vascular pedicle cannot be dealt with laparoscopically, the procedure should be rapidly converted.

Ensuring that the dissection is in the correct anatomical plane, which lies between the colonic mesentery and retroperitoneum, can prevent ureteric injury. It is imperative that the ureter is deemed to be clear when dividing the inferior mesenteric artery. For right colectomies, the ureter does not pose as much of a problem in comparison to the left colectomy, but the duodenum can be injured during hepatic flexure mobilisation. The energy source used for dissection should be cooled before it is used to handle bowel.

There should be a low threshold for postoperative diagnostic laparoscopy if an anastomotic leak is suspected. The transanal approach may be contemplated if the leak is posterior and amenable to suture repair.

## References

1. Dai WC, Ng KK, Chok KS, Cheung TT, Poon RT, Fan ST (2010) Radiofrequency ablation for controlling iatrogenic splenic injury. Int J Colorectal Dis 25:667–668
2. Mirnezami A, Mirnezami R, Chandrakumaran K, Sasapu K, Sagar P, Finan P (2011) Increased local recurrence and reduced survival from colorectal cancer following anastomotic leak: systematic review and meta-analysis. Ann Surg 253:890–898
3. Park JS, Choi GS, Kim SH, Kim HR, Kim NK, Lee KY, Kang SB, Kim JY, Lee KY, Kim BC, Bae BN, Son GM, Lee SI, Kang H (2013) Multicenter analysis of risk factors for anastomotic leakage after laparoscopic rectal cancer excision: the Korean laparoscopic colorectal surgery study group. Ann Surg 257:665–671
4. Slieker JC, Komen N, Mannaerts GH, Karsten TM, Willemsen P, Murawska M, Jeekel J, Lange JF (2012) Long-term and perioperative corticosteroids in anastomotic leakage: a prospective study of 259 left-sided colorectal anastomoses. Arch Surg 147:447–452
5. Lee WS, Yun SH, Roh YN, Yun HR, Lee WY, Cho YB, Chun HK (2008) Risk factors and clinical outcome for anastomotic leakage after total mesorectal excision for rectal cancer. World J Surg 32:1124–1129
6. Leichtle SW, Mouawad NJ, Welch KB, Lampman RM, Cleary RK (2012) Risk factors for anastomotic leakage after colectomy. Dis Colon Rectum 55:569–575
7. Post IL, Verheijen PM, Pronk A, Siccama I, Houweling PL (2012) Intraoperative blood pressure changes as a risk factor for anastomotic leakage in colorectal surgery. Int J Colorectal Dis 27:765–772
8. Zakrison T, Nascimento BA Jr, Tremblay LN, Kiss A, Rizoli SB (2007) Perioperative vasopressors are associated with an increased risk of gastrointestinal anastomotic leakage. World J Surg 31:1627–1634
9. Schietroma M, Carlei F, Cecilia EM, Piccione F, Bianchi Z, Amicucci G (2012) Colorectal infraperitoneal anastomosis: the effects of perioperative supplemental oxygen administration on the anastomotic dehiscence. J Gastrointest Surg 16:427–434
10. Geiger TM, Horst S, Muldoon R, Wise PE, Enrenfeld J, Poulose B, Herline AJ (2012) Perioperative core body temperatures effect on outcome after colorectal resections. Am Surg 78:607–612
11. Titu LV, Tweedle E, Rooney PS (2008) High tie of the inferior mesenteric artery in curative surgery for left colonic and rectal cancers: a systematic review. Dig Surg 25:148–157
12. Bonnet S, Berger A, Hentati N, Abid B, Chevallier JM, Wind P, Delmas V, Douard R (2012) High tie versus low tie vascular ligation of the inferior mesenteric artery in colorectal cancer surgery: impact on the gain in colon length and implications on the feasibility of anastomoses. Dis Colon Rectum 55:515–521

13. Gadiot RP, Dunker MS, Mearadji A, Mannaerts GH (2011) Reduction of anastomotic failure in laparoscopic colorectal surgery using antitraction sutures. Surg Endosc 25:68–71
14. Lane JC, Wright S, Burch J, Kennedy RH, Jenkins JT (2013) Early prediction of adverse events in enhanced recovery based upon the host systemic inflammatory response. Colorectal Dis 15:224–230
15. Kornmann VN, Treskes N, Hoonhout LH, Bollen TL, van Ramshorst B, Boerma D (2012) Systematic review on the value of CT scanning in the diagnosis of anastomotic leakage after colorectal surgery. Int J Colorectal Dis 28(4):437–445

# Laparoscopic Spleen Surgery: Procedure, Complications, Reoperations and Tips and Tricks

# 5

Selman Uranues and R. Latifi

**Key Points**

- The treatment of splenic diseases has changed over the past decade, particularly for trauma, from prompt splenectomy in most cases to splenic salvage whenever possible. The most important factors influencing this change are the recognition that the majority of splenic traumas (grades I–IV) can be managed nonoperatively and the risk of infection after splenectomy.
- The spleen is the most important peripheral immune organ and contains more lymphatic tissue than all the lymph nodes in the human body taken together. The spleen is connected to the circulatory system and plays a central role in the immune system.
- If the spleen is to continue to fulfil its immunological functions, about 25 % of the original weight of a normal-sized organ should be available for preservation, along with adequate arterial blood supply.
- Laparoscopic splenectomy is mainly indicated for haematological disorders and only rarely for trauma.
- A partial resection of the spleen may be necessary with benign lesions (cysts, hamartoma, etc.) limited to one pole or half of the organ or for diagnostic purposes if other diagnostic measures have not secured a diagnosis.

**Electronic supplementary material** The online version of this chapter (doi:10.1007/978-3-319-19623-7_5) contains supplementary material, which is available to authorized users.

S. Uranues, MD, FACS (✉)
Section for Surgical Research, Department of Surgery, Medical University of Graz,
Auenbruggerplatz 29, 8036 Graz, Austria
e-mail: selman.uranues@medunigraz.at

R. Latifi, MD, FACS, FICS
Professor of Surgery, University of Arizona, Tucson, Arizona, USA

- Anatomical and technical considerations are important safety prerequisites in splenic surgery. The spleen can be considered to have two separate blood supplies:
  - (a) The main blood supply from the splenic artery and vein and their branches
  - (b) Supplemental blood circulation through the vessels in the ligaments
- The three major aims during splenic surgery are:
  - (a) Definitive anatomical dissection of the vessels, avoiding pancreatic injury
  - (b) Avoiding and controlling active haemorrhage
  - (c) Partial resection that preserves as much of the spleen as possible
- The three major complications during or after splenic surgery are:
  - (a) Bleeding
  - (b) Pancreatitis and pancreatic fistula
  - (c) Infections
- Patients who have undergone splenectomy should be informed of their immune deficit and vaccinated against pneumococci.

## 5.1    Problem

The most important problem during spleen surgery is bleeding, from the hilar vessels or the splenic parenchyma itself; it can occur at any stage of the operation and may be difficult to stop. Peri- and postoperative bleeds occur in up to 10 % of cases and depend on concomitant diseases and risk factors. Patients with haematological diseases and/or anticoagulant therapy are at greater risk; portal hypertension is a further risk factor.

Injuries to neighbouring organs, such as the flexure of the left colon and especially the tail of the pancreas, are far less common but pose serious complications. Postoperative pancreatitis can follow an injury, but blood supply to the tail of the pancreas may be compromised by proximal ligature of the splenic vessels, causing necrosis and possible formation of persisting fistulas.

Key elements for complication-free splenic surgery are knowledge of the surgical anatomy and laparoscopic expertise, as well as adherence to preventive measures and to the step-by-step dissection techniques.

## 5.2    Surgical Anatomy of the Spleen

For its size, the spleen is very well perfused. It is a soft lymphatic organ and contains about 1/4 of the body's total lymphoid tissue, but unlike the lymph nodes, it is integrated into the blood rather than lymphatic circulatory system. The hilum of the spleen is located roughly in the middle of the visceral surface, where the branches of the splenic artery enter and the tributaries of the splenic vein leave. This is the only place where it is not covered by the peritoneum. The spleen is suspended in the left upper quadrant by the splenophrenic, gastrosplenic and splenocolic ligaments; its physiological position and its shape can vary according to the position and distension of the neighbouring organs and the position of the body.

Generally the splenic artery has one branch each to the upper and lower poles and itself enters the spleen in the middle of the hilum so that the spleen can be divided into three segments: upper, middle and lower. These segments are quite autonomous in their arterial and venous circulation. The segments are superposed perpendicularly along the long axis of the spleen and are separated by poorly vascularised planes. The splenic branches are considered to be nonanastomosing terminal arteries, except for some intrahilar shunts; there are also a few intersegmental vessels that allow subtotal permeation of the segments with an increase in pressure. Intersegmental connections allow ligature of the main vessel or a catheter embolisation, which is usually be tolerated without total necrosis. Thanks to these poorly vascularised intersegmental zones, the spleen can be partially resected with minimal blood loss.

Based on the distribution of blood vessels within the splenic parenchyma, we distinguish between a central zone near the hilum, a peripheral zone distant from the hilum and an intermediate zone between the two. Understanding these zones of vascularisation is important for classifying the severity of splenic injuries, particularly intraoperative injuries. An intraoperative injury that involves only peripheral (subcapsular) parenchyma opens the peripheral arterioles and venous sinuses. The trabecular vessels are affected in the intermediate area. Parenchymal injuries of the medial surface penetrating into the central zone often damage the segmental vessels. Surgical measures are determined by the nature and degree of vascular injuries.

## 5.3 Diagnosis of the Complications

### 5.3.1 Bleeding

Intraoperative bleeding is not difficult to diagnose, but small vascular injuries may not be recognised intraoperatively and only become apparent postoperatively. They can be best diagnosed on the basis of laboratory work (CBC), cardiocirculatory parameters (clinically) and ultrasound. Drains are only reliable when there is considerable haemorrhagic output, but a drain with no output is by no means a guarantee that there is no bleeding. A diagnostic CT scan for postoperative bleeding is needed only rarely, if at all, in complex cases.

### 5.3.2 Injury to the Tail of Pancreas

Intraoperative injuries to the tail of the pancreas are infrequent but can be serious, particularly if not recognised intraoperatively. They occur in patients with difficult anatomy and when there is a poor view, in obese patients and in those with spleno-megaly, enlarged hilar lymph nodes and kyphosis. These injuries occur most often in the course of a total splenectomy; with partial splenectomy, there is little likeli-hood of a pancreas injury due to the anatomical distance. Commonly, injuries to the pancreas become clinically apparent during the postoperative course, with symp-toms resembling pancreatitis. If a drain is in place, amylase and lipase can be detected in the drain fluid, but it is clinically important only when the levels exceed the serum value by a factor of three. Besides the clinical course, CT is the most use-ful diagnostic method and will guide the management when there is a fluid collec-tion that requires drainage. Small injuries to the tail of pancreas usually do not cause complications and heal spontaneously, though they can also lead to clinically rele-vant fistulas.

The clinical effects of a postoperative pancreatic fistula are graded from A to C.

### 5.3.2.1 Grade A

The patient is clinically unremarkable, without persistent fistula or abdominal fluid collection. Diagnosis is made with CT. There is no therapeutic consequence and, in general, the hospital stay is not prolonged.

### 5.3.2.2 Grade B

These patients are symptomatic but stable, requiring diagnostic evaluation and ther-apeutic intervention. The patient may complain of abdominal pain, fever, nausea, intolerance of oral intake and bowel-related symptoms.

The fluid collection measures at least $3 \times 3$ cm by CT or ultrasound (US). Therapeutic interventions are antibiotics and enteral nutrition past the ligament of Treitz or parenteral nutrition. The drain should remain in place until the fistula has healed. Invasive intervention (CT-guided drainage) may be necessary and the hospi-tal stay is usually prolonged.

### 5.3.2.3 Grade C

Clinically unstable patient (sepsis) requiring intensive care. Therapeutic interven-tions are percutaneous drainage or re-laparotomy if the drain has become dislocated or is not optimally positioned; haemorrhage is common and high mortality is expected.

Postoperative pancreatic fistula (PPF) after splenectomy is a rare but dreaded and sometimes fatal postoperative surgical complication. The PPF after splenec-tomy can have serious consequences for the patient (readmission, reoperation, radiologically guided percutaneous drainage, prolonged parenteral antibiotics, numerous follow-up visits) and the related public health costs. Inflammation and sepsis, often associated with such fistulas, are responsible for metabolic disturbances that can culminate in multiorgan failure. Complications and their sequelae can only be prevented with perfect planning and excellent execution of the operation, whereby the importance of careful dissection cannot be overemphasised.

## 5.3.3    Positioning of the Patient During Laparoscopic Splenectomy

For laparoscopic splenectomy, the position of the patient is at least as important as the choice of trocar sites. The patient is positioned in a right semilateral position with the left arm fixed over the head. This permits a better approach to the spleen via the left thoracic aperture. In this position, the spleen hangs from its dorsolateral ligaments and the other organs shift caudally to expose the splenic hilum.

### 5.3.3.1 Trocar Placement

Three to four trocars are appropriate in most cases. The trocar placement should be chosen carefully on the basis of the size of the spleen. The first trocar is inserted in the umbilical region using an open technique and serves as the camera port. A 12-mm trocar is inserted next on the left medioclavicular line, either cranially or caudally from the level of the umbilicus, depending on the size of the spleen. It serves as the working trocar through which the endostapler is introduced to ligate the splenic vessels. The third is a 5-mm trocar, placed in the epigastric region; it is the second working trocar and is used exclusively to introduce a grasper or a suction device. These three trocars generally suffice. In exceptional cases, a fourth 5-mm trocar can be inserted for a retractor.

## 5.3.4    Operative Procedure

### 5.3.4.1 First Step: Mobilisation

Dissection is usually performed from the caudal to cranial direction with gentle dissection of the omentum from the lower pole and visceral aspect and/or splenic hilum. It is important to dissect close to the spleen but without tearing the capsule. In this phase, the short gastric vessels are also severed. The spleen is dissected and mobilised with ultrasonic scissors or a LigaSure® instrument exclusively, avoiding the use of clips and reducing changes of instruments to allow faster and safer dissection.

When the omental attachments on the medial surface and the short gastric and lower pole vessels have been severed, dorsolateral mobilisation can start with severing of the peritoneal fold. Dorsolateral mobilisation should only be done when all the connections on the visceral side have been severed as the dorsolateral fixation holds the spleen in its natural position and prevents it from falling into the medial surgical field. During this phase, great attention should be paid to the tail of the pancreas, which should be treated with utmost care and not injured. Blood supply to the tail of the pancreas by the last branches of the splenic and gastroepiploic vessels should by all means be preserved.

### 5.3.4.2 Second Step: Dissection of the Hilar Vessels

The hilar vessels should be dissected cleanly and are best transected with an endostapler. With this instrument, even large arteries and congested vessels can be ligated safely. Depending on the size of the hilum, a 45–60-mm vascular cartridge is usually suitable and assures safe closure of the splenic vessels.

### 5.3.4.3 Third Step: Prevention of Bleeding

The use of haemostatic substances such as collagen fleece and/or fibrin glue has proved to be valuable when there is a pronounced bleeding tendency, as, for example with hepatic cirrhosis, coagulopathies and thrombocytopenia. A suitable laparoscopic device is used routinely to spray the entire splenic fossa with fibrin sealant (Tisseel^R, Baxter) and tamponade the stumps of the blood vessels and the edge of the pancreatic tail with collagen fleece (TissuFleece^R or Hemopatch^R, Baxter). Only in exceptional cases is it necessary to drain the splenic fossa; when it is, the drain is removed on the second postoperative day at the latest.

## 5.4    Partial Splenectomy

### 5.4.1    Positioning of the Patient and the Trocar Placement

As for a laparoscopic total splenectomy, for hemisplenectomy the patient is placed on the operating table in a right semilateral position. The positions of the trocars other than the umbilical optic trocar differ, with a 5-mm trocar placed in the medioclavicular line; the epigastric trocar has a diameter of 12 mm. For the transsection of the splenic parenchyma, the endostapler is inserted from the medial direction via the 12-mm trocar port on the epigastrium and not caudally as when the splenic vessels are severed for a total splenectomy.

### 5.4.2    First Step: Mobilisation

For the partial resection, the dissection begins with mobilisation of only that part of the spleen that is to be resected. If the lower half of the spleen is to be removed, the omental attachments including the branches of the gastroepiploic artery are first severed using ultrasonic scissors or the LigaSure® instrument.

If the upper half is to be removed, mobilisation begins with the medial surface at the intended line for parenchymal transsection above the entrance of the main vessels. After the short gastric vessels have been severed, the peritoneal fold is dissected dorsal to the spleen, completing the mobilisation of the half of the spleen that is to be removed.

### 5.4.3    Second Step: Vascular Dissection

The vessels of the part of the spleen that is to be removed are severed gently and carefully, either by mechanical coagulation or stapler transection. This is the step with the highest risk of intraoperative bleeding and must be completed carefully.

Bleeding from the spleen is usually due to a capsular tear from tension on attachments or small vessels entering the spleen. Immediate pressure and coagulation with LigaSure® or ultrasonic scissors will usually stop the bleeding.

### 5.4.4 Third Step: Parenchymal Resection

With few exceptions, the parenchyma can be transected with an endostapler using a 60-mm parenchymal cartridge. The parenchyma is first compressed with a long, atraumatic grasper on the planned transection line that the previous vascular dissection has rendered clearly visible. To avoid tearing the capsule and causing bleeding, compression should be applied slowly and stepwise. Only when the parenchyma has been sufficiently compressed is it stapled through the epigastric 12-mm trocar and the resection performed, usually in two or more steps depending on the size of the organ.

### 5.4.5 Fourth Step: Securing the Resected Edge and Removal of the Specimen

The cut edge of the remaining portion of the spleen is sealed, preferably with a fibrin glue (Tisseel, Baxter) and collagen fleece (TissuFleece) or covered with a Hemopatch® (Baxter) to prevent afterbleeding. Both the fibrin adhesive and the collagen fleece help the spleen adhere to its surroundings quickly and so reduce the likelihood of torsion or buckling, especially in the venous area.

## 5.5 Haemostasis in Laparoscopic Spleen Surgery

Haemostasis is one of the greatest challenges in laparoscopic surgery. There can be bleeding with both uneventful and eventful laparoscopies. Scars and adhesions can change the anatomy and complicate dissection. The bleeding risk is also higher in patients with abnormal tissue characteristics due to medications such as cortisone, thrombocyte aggregation inhibitors or anticoagulants.

Bleeding resulting from intraoperative developments and difficulties is usually due to inadequate exposure or inability to manipulate the tissue or to equipment failure.

With all these possible causes of bleeding, the most important thing is prevention.

This means that the surgeon must be alert to the fact that there can always be anatomical variations and must ensure that the correct instrument or dissection device is used. It must be borne in mind that all the high-tech devices nonetheless have their pitfalls and do not always and in every case have the same safety characteristics. Vessels with a diameter of 5 mm or more should be dissected with the LigaSure® or other ultrasonic dissector or with an endostapler.

Even with all preventive measures in place, there can still be bleeding. To manage it, the following materials should be available in the operating room and not have to be fetched from somewhere else. Most important are sutures for laparoscopy, endoloops, collagen fleece and fibrin adhesive. Before the procedure is begun, the team should discuss what is to be done in the case of acute bleeding.

Fast and effective haemostasis is only possible when the source of the bleeding is visible. This means that with spurting blood, the person operating the camera should, without losing the view, quickly retract the trocar a few millimetres to prevent loss of vision. As the very first measure, simple pressure or pinching can temporarily stop the bleeding and let the team calm down. Before final haemostasis can be achieved, the source of the bleeding will usually need to be dissected free for better visibility. To this end, the operating surgeon should best use his/her nondominant hand to keep the bleeding under control and perform the other manipulations with the dominant hand. For venous bleeds, compression with a small sponge introduced into the abdominal cavity through a 10-mm trocar works best. Arteries with a diameter of up to 7 mm can be sealed with a modern coagulation device, an endoloop or a clip, but venous bleeds require suturing. In advanced laparoscopy, the operating surgeon should have perfect mastery of laparoscopic suturing and intracorporal knotting techniques. After a manoeuvre of this sort, the tail of the pancreas and other neighbouring organs should be inspected for accidental injuries. Spurting arterial bleeds require surgical haemostasis by coagulation or suture. Parenchymal bleeds can be stopped very simply and effectively with FloSeal. Oozing from the spleen can be stopped effectively and once and for all with a Hemopatch® or with compression followed by tamponade with collagen fleece using fibrin adhesive. Before a haemostyptic is applied, compression should be applied patiently as long as necessary.

With complicated procedures, it is usually advantageous to use a drain, preferably an active suction drain which, however, should not be located near the source of bleeding.

## Further Reading

Targarona EM, Gracia E, Rodriguez M, Cerdan G, Balague C, Garriga J, Trias M (2003) Hand-assisted laparoscopic surgery. Arch Surg 138:133–141

Uranues S, Alimoglu O (2005) Laparoscopic surgery of the spleen. Surg Clin North Am 85(1):75–90, ix. Review

Uranues S, Grossman D, Ludwig L, Bergamaschi R (2007) Laparoscopic partial splenectomy. Surg Endosc 21(1):57–60, Epub 9 Oct 2006

Uranüs S, Pfeifer J, Schauer C, Kronberger L Jr, Rabl H, Ranftl G, Hauser H, Bahadori K (1995) Laparoscopic partial splenic resection. Surg Laparosc Endosc 5:133–136

# Complications After Total Endoscopic Preperitoneal (TEP) Repair

# 6

Salvador Morales-Conde

## 6.1 Introduction

Complications of laparoscopic surgery are different from those of conventional surgery. Laparoscopy seems to repair inguinal hernias with a lower rate of postoperative complications, especially to those related to surgical wound morbidity, infections or bleeding events, and postoperative surgical pain, but always these complications depend on the surgeon's experience. Furthermore, the type and size of the hernia along with the patient's conditions will also influence the presence of complications. On the other hand, most of intraoperative complications associated with this technique include complications due to the laparoscopic access, such as trocar injuries, although many specific complications related to the dissection of the area, mesh placement and fixation have also been described.

Laparoscopic surgery in inguinal hernia is associated to a complete change of the vision of the anatomy vs. conventional approach that adds technical difficulty, especially in the TEP (total extraperitoneal), where working space is limited and manoeuvres dissections are more complex.

In laparoscopic repair of inguinal hernias, there are two techniques well differentiated: total extraperitoneal approach (TEP) and transabdominal preperitoneal approach (TAPP), the intraoperative complications of each of them are differents. For this reason, it is important to describe complications specifically related to each technique.

**Electronic supplementary material** The online version of this chapter (doi:10.1007/978-3-319-19623-7_6) contains supplementary material, which is available to authorized users.

S. Morales-Conde
Unit of Innovation in Minimally Invasive Surgery, Department of Surgery, University Hospital "Virgen del Rocío", Sevilla, Spain
e-mail: smoralesc@gmail.com

## 6.2    Intraoperative Complications Related to TEP

### 6.2.1    Complications Related to the Access to the Preperitoneal Space

These complications are frequent during the learning curve and may force conversion to an open surgical technique. One of the main steps of this technique includes the access to the preperitoneal space. Inadequate access may lead to conversion to TAPP or to open surgery.

Access to this space may be carried out by blunt dissection, assisted by the tip of the optic followed by dissection with one instrument after introduction of the first trocar, or using a balloon. A randomised, prospective, multicentre study showed that a dissection balloon made the dissection of the preperitoneal space easier and safer, thus reducing operative time, conversion rate and number of complications.

Complications related to access to the preperitoneal space include:

1. *Problems related to epigastric vessels*:
   (a) Blunt dissection with the finger before introduction of the trocar could lead to a tear of the epigastric vessels, resulting in intense bleeding. To avoid bleeding, it is important to introduce the finger below the rectus muscle without doing any lateral movement.
   (b) Another problem related to epigastric vessels includes dissection of the vessels from the anterior wall during dissection of the preperitoneal space, which makes surgery more difficult. It is important to perform a proper blunt dissection with the finger and to visualise the epigastric vessel through the balloon during insufflation, by introducing the optic inside of it, in order to guarantee that epigastric vessels are maintained attached to the anterior wall.
2. *Problems related to balloon dissection*: Besides the problems previously mentioned, bleeding of the epigastric vessels, peritoneal tears could also be related to balloon dissection. Smooth insufflation of the balloon is one of the main steps to avoid this problem. On the other hand, proper indications for access and for the technique itself are other factors to avoid peritoneal tears. Patients with previous infraumbilical surgery could present fibrous tissue in this space with a difficult distension of the preperitoneal area. In this case, it is even more important to have slow and little dissection of the space with the balloon, continuing the dissection using scissors through the 5-mm trocar. In case of midline infraumbilical surgery, the incision for introduction of the balloon should be performed laterally to the incision, through the rectus muscle. In case of previous surgery in the preperitoneal space, such us prostatectomy, TAPP could be a better indication, although different authors, such as Dulucq et al., have shown that it is feasible. The last advice to avoid complications during balloon dissection include the recommendation of not to insufflate the balloon more than it is accepted, since it could blow up and make a massive tear of the peritoneum with the subsequent need to collect the different plastic parts of the balloon.

3. *Visceral and vascular injuries*: These complications could happen during insertion of trocars to perform surgery. Since there is no access to the abdominal cavity, visceral injuries due to introduction of trocars are very rare in this approach.

4. *Bladder injuries*: The most common visceral injury during TEP is related to injury of the bladder, while bowel injuries are uncommon, as trocars are inserted when the preperitoneal space is already created and under direct vision. Injury to the bladder has been reported in 8 of 3868 patients who underwent surgery during a 7.5-year period, the majority of whom had previously undergone suprapubic catheterisation. Laparoscopic peritoneal access or secondary suprapubic trocar placement can result in a bladder perforation, usually as result of failure to decompress a distended bladder. Less commonly, the injury is associated with a congenital bladder abnormality. Aspects to be considered to prevent or to treat this complication are:

   (a) A proper indication of the hernia to be repaired is an important factor to avoid this complication. Those cases with previous surgery in the preperitoneal space, such as prostatectomy, could increase adhesions of the bladder in this space, increasing the possibility of having an injury, especially during the manoeuvres of dissection of the preperitoneal space. Bladder is especially prone to injury during laparoscopic inguinal hernia repair when the preperitoneal space has previously been dissected, e.g. previous preperitoneal hernia repair or prostatectomy. Incarcerated hernias could also be related to these injuries, since the hernia sac is not yet reduced when the preperitoneal space is being created and a trocar may be inserted into the bladder. Based on this, correct indications for surgery are the best way to avoid this complication. Even though some authors have demonstrated good results with this approach in patients with previous prostatectomy, these hernias should be performed by TAPP approach, especially if surgeons are not experienced with this other technique.

   (b) Special mention should be made to large direct or medial hernias, since the bladder can be a frequent content of this type of hernias and usually the sac is attached to the transversalis fascia when the space is created. On the other hand, caution must be taken when reducing this sac, as improper traction can result in injury.

   (c) Another aspect to be considered is when hernia repair is performed in a patient with the bladder filled with urine. In this case, the bladder can decrease the preperitoneal space and trocars become more prone to injure the bladder. For this reason, it is recommended to have the patient emptying the bladder before going to operating room.

   (d) This lesion shall be suspected if urine is withdrawn into a syringe after Veress needle insertion or if blood and gas are noticed in the urine drainage bag if the patient is catheterised. In questionable cases, methylene blue dye may be instilled into the bladder to look for leakage. Bladder injury recognised during laparoscopy shall be repaired laparoscopically, providing the experience of the surgeon is sufficient. This should be followed by bladder drainage for 7–10 days.

(e) Bladder injury may present in a delayed fashion with haematuria and lower abdominal discomfort. Contrast-enhanced computerised tomography, cystography, or cystoscopy are the primary imaging techniques used to evaluate patients for suspected injury. Small defects may be managed with postoperative decompression via an indwelling catheter for urinary drainage, whereas larger defects need repair.

5. *Trocar site hernias*: Hernias at trocar site are very rare after TEP for different reasons: first reason is because assisting trocars are usually 5-mm trocars, and the second reason is that the 10–12-mm trocars just open the anterior fascia, maintaining the posterior fascia of the rectus muscle preserved.

6. *Hypercapnia*: This complication occurs during $CO_2$ insufflation. The absorption of $CO_2$ in the preperitoneal space is higher than intraperitoneally, being a factor to be considered when insufflation of $CO_2$ happens in a virtual space, especially preperitoneally. This complication is related in most cases to the learning curve, since longer intraoperative time can increase the absorption of $CO_2$ by blood vessels of the preperitoneal space. Expert surgeons with short surgical time rarely see this complication, as it can be prevented by decreasing surgical time. On the other hand, the role of the anaesthesiologist is very important in order to monitor this situation.

7. *Subcutaneous emphysema*: This complication is common, but does not require any treatment, since $CO_2$ is rapidly absorbed right after surgery.

## 6.2.2  Complications Related to the Dissection of the Hernia

1. *Bowel injury*: Studies on TEP and TAPP report intraoperative intestinal injury in 0–0.3 % of cases, with rates of 0–0.06 % in larger investigations involving over 1000 patients. Problems can arise if patients are not correctly placed in the Trendelenburg position. When this happens, the intestines can remain in the hernia sac, increasing the risk of thermal damage. Extraperitoneal laparoscopic surgery is performed under general anaesthesia with good muscle relaxation, otherwise the working space is too small and the bowel would be pushing the preperitoneal space, increasing the risk of injury. On the other hand, in case there is any gas leak, the preperitoneal space also becomes too small. For this reason, we use the balloon trocar to make the incision airtight.

2. *Vascular injuries*: In large investigations, involving over 1000 patients, the rates of injuries to great vessels are of 0–0.11 %. These vascular injuries may arise from injury to major vessels, to epigastric vessels, to vessels from the cord or to vessels surrounding Cooper's ligament. During dissection, the surgeon must visualise an aspect of "spider's web", to indicate that he/she is in the right direction. Dissection must be blunt in order to decrease the possibility of an injury to the vessels of this space. During this dissection, the surgeon uses diathermy to control possible bleeding from small vessels. The bipolar method seems to be safer than the monopolar. Different situations, besides bleeding of epigastric vessels which have been previously described, are:

(a) At the high end of the dissection, there is always a small vessel, collateral of the inferior epigastric vessels. This vessel has to be coagulated with diathermy to prevent bleeding.

(b) The vas deferens is seen lying separately on the medial side, and the gonadal vessels are seen laterally, forming a triangle. This triangle, known as the "triangle of doom", is bounded medially by the vans deferens, laterally by the gonadal vessels, with its apex at the internal inguinal ring, and the base is formed by the peritoneum. Dissection should be clear in this region, to avoid injury to the cord structures or iliac vessels.

(c) Bleeding from the vessels surrounding the area of the Cooper's ligament might be difficult to control, being most of the time controlled with precise coagulation. In case of difficulty to control bleeding, the best methods to achieve a good haemostasis are to introduce gauze and to compress or to use some haemostatic agents.

(d) Injury to the major vessels can be fatal and usually requires urgent laparotomy and vascular repair.

3. *Peritoneal tears*: During dissection of the peritoneum, breaches in it can be found. Peritoneal tear is the most common reason for conversion and predisposes patients to small-bowel adhesions and internal herniation. The mesh will no longer be securely buttressed between the abdominal wall and retroperitoneum by intra-abdominal pressure and becomes susceptible to migrate if not stapled. Hence, closure of the defect is preferred. The following aspects must be considered:

(e) The presence of a previous mesh from a prior hernia repair presents a technical challenge for TAPP or TEP repairs of recurrence. The mesh from a prior Lichtenstein repair should not affect the field of a posterior approach. The best approach to a mesh placed during prior laparoscopic repairs may be to leave it in place, avoiding the risk of injury to the iliac vein or to the bladder. The new mesh can be laid on top of the old one to correct technical failures of a slipped or misplaced previously placed mesh. However, the mesh plug technique poses a unique problem for a laparoscopic repair of recurrence. The old plug creates an obstacle for dissection of the preperitoneal space, creating conditions to produce tears of it, and, on the other hand, can also be an obstacle to place the new mesh and to replace the peritoneum over it. Removal of the plug is not simple and cannot be easily accomplished with endo-shears. We find that electrocautery more effectively cuts the protruding aspect of the plug, thus allowing the possibility of posterior mesh placement and replacement and repair of the peritoneum. For this reason, the best approach for a recurrent hernia after plug technique is a TAPP, since the peritoneum can be more easily dissected from the plug than using a TEP approach.

(f) The TEP technique must be meticulous and all peritoneum openings have to be closed to prevent postoperative occlusion. An Endoloop® is usually used to close those breaches in the peritoneum. If the peritoneal tear is near the arched line, the scope could be moved down, changing the 10-mm optic to a 5-mm one, to facilitate triangulation. If the closure is impossible, the surgeon should change to TAPP or to open procedure. If a pneumoperitoneum ensues, a Veress needle can be placed in the left hypochondrium to reduce it, increasing the space in the preperitoneal area. If there is doubt about a peritoneal breach, the procedure shall be completed with a laparoscopic exploration to investigate the pelvis. If there is a gap, it can be closed with sutures.

4. *Difficult reduction of incarcerated hernias*: In 2004, Ferzli et al. described their experience with TEP in repairing 11 acutely incarcerated inguinal hernias. Eight repairs were completed via TEP, and three converted to open repairs. They describe the use of various releasing incisions to free the incarcerated sac depending on the nature of the hernia (direct, indirect or femoral). This author reported no recurrences, a single mesh infection that resolved with continuous irrigation and a midline wound infection after bowel resection. In 2003, Tamme et al. showed their results in a large series of TEP repairs of inguinal hernias. In this group, they include, but does not detail, repairs performed on strangulated hernias. Their overall results demonstrated low rates of recurrence and complications. Amongst their conclusions, there is the statement that TEP is particularly advantageous for the treatment of bilateral, recurrent and strangulated hernias vs. open and TAPP repairs. They cite a reduction in postoperative neuralgia vs. open repair and a reduction in bowel injury and port site hernia vs. TAPP. Saggar and Sarang retrospectively looked at 34 patients (of 286 elective TEP hernia repairs) who underwent repair of chronically incarcerated inguinal hernia using TEP. Recurrence rate was higher for incarcerated vs. nonincarcerated hernias (5.8 vs. 0.35 %). Recurrences in the incarcerated group ($n = 2$) occurred during the immediate postoperative period and 2 months postoperatively. Scrotal haematoma and cord induration also were significantly higher in the incarcerated group. They converted the umbilical port to an intraperitoneal one to inspect the bowel when its viability was in question. Besides the good results published in repairing incarcerated hernias, TAPP seems to be the preferable option to repair these types of hernias, as hernia contents are easily controlled with the intraperitoneal vision, the operation, in these cases, being, thus, safer.

5. *Problems related to large sac*: In a case of indirect hernia, lateral to the inferior epigastric vessels, the peritoneal sac is dissected away from cord structures, both medially and laterally until it is completely separated and then dealt with appropriately. At times, a long indirect sac cannot be completely reduced from the deep inguinal ring and is divided, with the peritoneal side being ligated with a laparoscopic suture. Laparoscopic repair of a scrotal hernia is a controversial subject in laparoscopy, because it implies a large abdominal wall defect and great difficulty in dissecting the extensive hernia sac. Literature on the subject is scant.

## 6.3 Postoperative Complications

1. *Haematoma at the hernia site*: Haematomas and seromas are most frequent complications, especially in the treatment of large indirect hernias (2–7 %). Usually they resolve spontaneously in about 6 weeks but may persist for several

months. They do not represent a problem for the patient to return to normal activity but must be identified and not confused with possible recurrences. When in doubt, ultrasound and time will confirm the diagnosis (the haematoma decreases their size and hardens, leaving a well-defined mass, and is painless). Some authors recommend routine use of a drain, because the release of carbon dioxide pressure is followed by bleeding from tiny capillaries, resulting in an unpredictable amount of blood collecting in the preperitoneal space. Furthermore, drainage also ensures complete deflation and readaptation of the tissue layer. Avoidance of postoperative haematomas is important to the achievement of a low mesh infection rate and prevention of potential mesh displacement because of the collected fluid. Even though drains might be useful to control this complication, correct haemostasis is the best way to prevent it, since drains can be a factor that influence the postoperative course of patients, producing an uncomfortable sensation which can delay hospital leave. On the other hand, authors that use fibrin glue to fix the mesh include it on their list of advantages; using this method of fixation, the haemostatic effect of the fibrin sealant is added, and this can decrease the presence of haematomas and ecchymosis in the area, resulting in better postoperative outcomes.

2. *Seroma*: Seroma is a frequent complication of endoscopic total extraperitoneal mesh repair of inguinal hernias, especially after a direct hernia, which may cause discomfort and anxiety. Its volume is proportional to the size of the preperitoneal "dead" space created after reduction of the hernia. Attempts to reduce its incidence after direct hernias have included tacking the transversalis fascia to the pubic ramus or closed suction drainage of the preperitoneal space. Both these techniques are not without problems. Primary closure of direct inguinal hernia defects with a pre-tied suture loop during endoscopic TEP repair is safe, efficient and very reliable for prevention of postoperative seroma formation, without increasing the risk of developing chronic groin pain or hernia recurrence. This technique should be the preferred method over stapling of transversalis fascia or insertion of a closed suction drainage device in such a situation.

3. *Infection*: Antibiotic prophylaxis in inguinal hernia surgery is controversial. Overall infection rate is low, with a mean value of 1–4 %. Infectious rate <2 % is regarded as a clean operation. Antibiotic prophylaxis may reduce wound infection rates with impact on patients' satisfaction, wound care and sick leave, but it also involves risks of toxicity, allergic side effects, bacterial resistance and higher costs. There has been a discussion on risk factors used to select the best candidates for antibiotic prophylaxis. Age >75 years, obesity and urinary catheter were heavy risk factors for global infectious complications in one study. Other known risk factors for infectious complications are hernia recurrence, diabetes, immune suppressants, corticosteroid usage and malignancy. Until now, a total of 14 RCTs comparing antibiotic prophylaxis vs. placebo in inguinal hernia surgery were identified, of which there was only 1 about laparoscopic repair and the remaining 13 were about open repair. The endoscopic RCT by Schwetling and Bärlehner has an incorrect randomisation, lacks

definition of wound infection and is heavily underpowered with only 40 patients in each arm. It does not allow any conclusions. For this reason, in other to avoid infection after TEP repair, the same protocol then after open inguinal hernia repair must be followed.

4. *Chronic pain*: Acute and chronic pain, defined as pain lasting for 3 months or more after inguinal hernia surgery, has emerged as a key issue in literature. Reported chronic pain rates after groin hernia repair vary from 0 to 75.5 %. Overall, moderate to severe pain was experienced by 10–12 % of patients. In this respect, operations performed endoscopically seem to be more favourable than both non-mesh and mesh open technique operations. A retrospective, multicentric comparison of 1972 TAPP and TEP hernia repairs using polyester meshes found no difference in chronic pain with rates of 0.6 and 0.7 % after TAPP and TEP, respectively. A systematic review of Wake et al. comparing TAPP and TEP showed no difference in early and chronic pain. According to the existing literature, there is no difference in acute and chronic pain after TAPP and TEP hernia repair. After introduction of endoscopic hernia surgery, mesh fixation was thought to be mandatory to avoid dislocation of the mesh and recurrences. Permanent fixation with tackers, staples or sutures was used. The perplexing problem of chronic pain after endoscopic hernia surgery raised the question of whether fixation is really necessary. Nerve entrapment and pain caused by shrinkage of the mesh due to scar tissue formation have been suggested as possible causes. As it can be observed, factors involved in chronic pain after TEP repair are fixation and type of mesh:

   (a) Fixation of mesh is typically performed to minimise risk of recurrence in laparoscopic inguinal hernia repair. Mesh fixation with staples has been implicated as a cause of chronic inguinal pain. Different studies have been performed to compare mesh fixation using fibrin sealant vs. staple fixation in laparoscopic inguinal hernia and to compare outcomes for hernia recurrence and chronic inguinal pain. Because fibrin glue mesh fixation in laparoscopic inguinal hernia repair achieves similar hernia recurrence rates compared with staple/tacker fixation, but decreased incidence of chronic inguinal pain, it may be the preferred technique. The technique of non-fixation or temporary fixation using glue is increasingly used to solve this pain problem

   (b) On the other hand, meshes might also have an influence in chronic pain. The last meta-analysis conducted by A Currie et al. in surgical endoscopy has shown that lightweight and heavyweight mesh repair had similar outcomes with regard to postoperative pain, seroma development and time to return to work after TEP repair.

5. *Nerve entrapment*: No injuries have been reported of the ilioinguinal or iliohypogastric nerve. Neuralgia paraesthetica may be originated due to the dissection or due to the fact of placing a tacker in the femoral cutaneous nerve causing injury or in femoral branch of the genitofemoral nerve. Anatomical knowledge of the preperitoneal space prevents such injuries, as well as non-fixation or glue fixation, as mentioned previously. The location of the staple by radiology and laparoscopic removal may solve the problem.

6. *Mesh-related complications*:
   (a) Migration of the mesh: This complication is related to insufficient fixation of the mesh to Cooper's ligament or to the use of a small size of prosthesis. To avoid this, one should always check the correct mesh placement and size. On the other hand, tears of the peritoneum, in those cases in which the mesh is not fixed, can be also related to mesh migration.
   (b) Infection: Rejection of the prosthesis, infection or retroperitoneal abscesses are rare. Recurrence does not usually happen if you need to remove the prosthesis.
   (c) Mesh erosion to the bladder: Mesh erosion to the bladder after laparoscopic inguinal hernia repair is rare; only eight cases have been reported since 1994. Therefore, the exact incidence is not known. Both polypropylene and expanded polytetrafluoroethylene have been incriminated. Probable causes are unrecognised injury to the bladder wall at the time of the laparoscopic inguinal hernia repair and improper placement of mesh and fixation material. Repeated urinary tract infections, haematuria or the development of bladder stones can all be presenting signs.
   (d) Adhesions and fistulas to intra-abdominal organs.
7. *Bowel obstruction*: This complication is caused by herniation of the small intestine through a peritoneal breach or by attachment of bowel to a missed peritoneal hole that could have enlarged in the postoperative period. Patients can go through laparoscopic revision, without need of intestinal resection. The risk of intestinal obstruction in the postoperative period is not more important for TEP than it is for Lichtenstein technique.
8. *Bowel perforation*: Perforations of small intestine in the postoperative period resulted from thermal injury during operation, and the symptoms manifest, usually, 5–8 days after surgery. During reoperation, by laparoscopy or laparotomy, there is no need to remove meshes, although local findings and the grade of the peritonitis can lead the surgeon to remove it.
9. *Urinary complications*: Urinary retention is less common after inguinal herniorrhaphies performed under local anaesthesia compared with general or regional one. However, this complication is more commonly related to spinal anaesthesia, which it is not usually used in laparoscopic approaches, but it also happens after general anaesthesia. The incidence varies widely from as low as 0.2 % in a single-author study from France to as high as 22.2 % of patients undergoing laparoscopic inguinal hernia repair in a study from Mayo Clinic in Rochester, Minnesota. More commonly, it is reported to occur in the 2–7 % range. Although reports in the literature conflict somewhat, in general older age, prostatic symptoms before surgery, postoperative use of narcotics and administration of postoperative intravenous fluid >500 cc have been found to be predictive. Type of procedure (TEP vs. TAPP), surgical time, anaesthesia time, intraoperative fluid restriction or development of other complications do not appear to be significant risk factors. In general, it can be avoided by restricting fluid intake, intraoperative and postoperative, and by early ambulation. If, after 8 h of surgery, the patient does not urinate spontaneously, bladder catheterisation shall be advised.

10. *Testicular complications*:
   (a) Transient postoperative pain: It is usually a burning testicular sensation due to trauma of the genitofemoral nerve or of the testicular sympathetic nerves or, still, to cord oedema, especially in case of fenestration of the mesh. It occurs in 0.2 % of cases. The discomfort is usually transient and responds to elevation of the testicle and analgesics.
   (b) Hydrocele: This complication appears in 1 % of the hernia repairs performed by laparoscopy, but the cause is not known. Whereas urological literature suggests that this is due to the practice of leaving the distal sac in situ, most experienced hernia surgeons do not accept this theory. Some authors propose that it occurs when an unrecognised vaginal process is blocked and the accumulated fluid cannot drain freely into the peritoneal cavity. It is important to differentiate hydrocele from seroma because the latter is almost always self-limiting and will resolve without treatment. The treatment is the same as for any other hydrocele.
   (c) Scrotal haematomas: This complication can be prevented after laparoscopic inguinal hernia repair if complete haemostasis is assured before completing the procedure. Conservative treatment (ice, scrotal support, pain management and observation) is sufficient for most, although large haematomas may require surgical drainage. Patients with bleeding disorders are especially prone to this complication.
   (d) Orchitis: It is defined as postoperative inflammation of the testicle occurring within 1–5 days after surgery. It is felt to be due to acute thrombosis of the delicate venous pampiniform plexus rather than arterial injury. It is most common after inguinal scrotal herniorrhaphy when extensive dissection of the spermatic cord has been performed. Presenting symptoms are low-grade fever with a painful and enlarged and firm testicle. The differential diagnosis includes scrotal haematoma and testicular torsion. Management is supportive with scrotal support and anti-inflammatory agents. Duplex ultrasound scanning is useful when infarction is suspected. Ischaemic orchitis may result in testicular necrosis within days or have a slower course resulting in testicular atrophy during a period of several months. Fortunately, most patients recover from ischaemic orchitis uneventfully without testicular atrophy. Interestingly, most patients who develop testicular atrophy do not provide history of orchitis. It is not yet known whether laparoscopy will have any advantage over conventional surgery because of the more proximal dissection in the preperitoneal space. However, in one large analysis of a prospectively maintained database containing 8050 TAPP laparoscopic hernia repairs, orchitis and testicular atrophy were reported to be extremely low at 0.1 and 0.05 %, respectively. Interestingly, this group removes all indirect sacs, no matter their size, except in rare circumstances of excessive inflammation. Nevertheless, based primarily on the extensive writings of the late George Wantz, undue dissection of cord and testicle to remove an indirect inguinal hernia sac completely is not recommended. The hernia sac can be divided at a conve-

nient point in the inguinal canal and has the distal aspect left open. The proximal sac is then dissected from the cord structures and ligated.

(e) Testicular atrophy: As it has been described, it is rare, even after injury of the spermatic vessels, due to the rich collateral circulation (0.3–0.5 % difference in classical surgery). Surgeon's experience makes this injury very rare after the initial learning curve, but it can be further avoided by minimising dissection of the cord and leaving the distal segment of the indirect sac.

11. *Sexual dysfunction and infertility*: In patients with inguinal hernias, sexual activity may be impaired due to hernia-related pain. Surgical repair may improve these complaints but can also lead to similar symptoms as long-term complication of the operation. Injury to the vas deferens can occur during laparoscopic inguinal hernia repair and, if bilateral, will lead to certain infertility. The vas deferens may be injured during dissection and mobilisation or during fixation of the mesh. Unilateral injury to the vas can lead to exposure of spermatozoa to the immune system and the formation of antisperm antibodies, causing secondary infertility. Bilateral testicular atrophy (discussed earlier) is another cause. A recent study that detailed 14 patients whose infertility was, apparently, the result of damage to the spermatic cord caused by normal fibroplastic response to polypropylene mesh, resulting in obstruction of the vas deferens included 10 open procedures, 2 laparoscopic and 2 where laparoscopy was used on one side and open on the other. However, the explanation for their findings might be a more traditional injury mechanism at time of surgery, such as ligation, division or cauterisation followed by scarring to the most convenient adjacent structure that, in this case, would be the mesh. Endoscopic hernia repair is associated with less postoperative pain and earlier return to normal activities, but its effect on pain-related sexual function has not been studied frequently. The study conducted by Schouten et al. shows that painful sexual activity is presented in one third of patients with inguinal hernias and is improved in the majority of patients following TEP hernia repair. Postoperatively, moderate to severe painful sexual activity occurred in 2.3 % of the patients with no history of preoperative complaints

## Further Reading

1. Kaul A, Hutfless S, Le H, Hamed SA, Tymitz K, Nguyen H, Marohn MR (2012) Staple versus fibrin glue fixation in laparoscopic total extraperitoneal repair of inguinal hernia: a systematic review and meta-analysis. Surg Endosc 26(5):1269–1278

2. Currie A, Andrew H, Tonsi A, Hurley PR, Taribagil S (2012) Lightweight versus heavyweight mesh in laparoscopic inguinal hernia repair: a meta-analysis. Surg Endosc 26(8):2126–2133

3. Schouten N, van Dalen T, Smakman N, Clevers GJ, Davids PH, Verleisdonk EJ, Tekatli H, Burgmans JP (2012) Impairment of sexual activity before and after endoscopic totally extraperitoneal (TEP) hernia repair. Surg Endosc 26(1):230–234

4. Bringman S, Ek A, Haglind E, Heikkinen T, Kald A, Kylberg F, Ramel S, Wallon C, Anderberg B (2001) Is a dissection balloon beneficial in totally extraperitoneal endoscopic hernioplasty (TEP)? A randomized prospective multicentre study. Surg Endosc 15:266–270

5. Chowbey P (2007) TEP. In: Fitzgibbons RJ, Schumpelick V (eds) Recurrent hernia. Prevention and treatment. Springer, Berlin, pp 274–279
6. Simons MP, Aufenacker T, Bay Nielsen M, Bouillot JL, Campanelli G, Conze J, de Lange D, Fortelny R, Heikkinen T, Kingsnorth A, Kukleta J, Morales-Conde S, Nordin P, Schumpelick V, Smedberg S, Smietanski M, Weber G, Miserez M (2009) European Hernia Society guidelines on the treatment of inguinal hernia in adult patients. Hernia 13:343–403
7. Lau H, Patil NG, Yuen WK, Lee F (2002) Management of peritoneal tear during endoscopic extraperitoneal inguinal hernioplasty. Surg Endosc 6:1474–1477
8. Moreno-Egea A et al (2004) Randomized clinical trial of fixation vs nonfixation mesh in total extraperitoneal inguinal hernioplasty. Arch Surg 139:1376–1379
9. Ferzli GS, Kiel T (1997) The role of the endoscopic extraperitoneal approach in large inguinal scrotal hernias. Surg Endosc 11:299–302
10. Eklund A et al (2007) Recurrent inguinal hernia: randomized multicenter trial comparing laparoscopic and Lichtenstein repair. Surg Endosc 21:634–640
11. Hamouda A, Kennedy J, Grant N, Nigam A, Karanjia N (2009) Mesh erosion into the urinary bladder following laparoscopic inguinal hernia repair; is this the tip of the iceberg? Hernia 14:314–349
12. Agrawal A, Avill R (2006) Mesh migration following repair of inguinal hernia: a case report and review of literature. Hernia 10:79–82
13. Winslow ER, Quasebarth M, Brunt LM (2004) Perioperative outcomes and complications of open vs laparoscopic extraperitoneal inguinal hernia repair in a mature surgical practice. Surg Endosc 18:221–227
14. Moore JB, Hasenboehler EA (2007) Orchiectomy as a result of ischemic orchitis after laparoscopic inguinal hernia repair: case report of a rare complication. Patient Saf Surg 1:3
15. Bittner R, Arregui ME, Bisgaard T, Dudai M, Ferzli GS, Fitzgibbons RJ, Fortelny RH, Klinge U, Kockerling F, Kuhry E, Kukleta J, Lomanto D, Misra MC, Montgomery A, Morales-Conde S, Reinpold W, Rosenberg J, Sauerland S, Schug-Pass C, Singh K, Timoney M, Weyhe D, Chowbey P (2011) Guidelines for laparoscopic (TAPP) and endoscopic (TEP) treatment of inguinal hernia [International Endohernia Society (IEHS)]. Surg Endosc 25(9):2773–2843. doi:10.1007/s00464-011-1799-6. Epub 2011 Jul 13

# Complications in TAPP Hernia Repair

# 7

Jan F. Kukleta

One should learn not only from his own errors, but from all errors of all others too.

Well-being is in general the expected outcome after any surgical intervention.

Both physicians and patients but even more the public opinion find any deviation from the expected "restitutio ad integrum" as something that went wrong: a complication. The so-called "adverse event" is often held for a result of incorrect or incompetent performance especially since medicine became a popular public matter.

Complication in surgery is an undesired disadvantageous deviation of an expected course.

The true incidence of complications in laparoscopic hernia repair is certainly underreported.

Hernia repair as one of the most frequent elective interventions in surgery is a very good example: the so-called simple operation that any surgeon can perform, an operation which represents the first steps in everyone's surgical education can cause so many unthinkable circumstances that may deteriorate the patient's quality of life. The unmet expectations fed by social media information burden the patient-doctor relationship. Parallel to the obvious progress in "hernia affairs", the subject became more complex. Introduction of new suture materials, meshes, improved visualisation, minimal invasive philosophy, miniaturisation of instruments, new approaches and new techniques have enabled a significant improvement of outcomes of today's hernia patients.

An experienced well-trained surgeon is aware of the permanent risk of complication in any act that he or she performs. Still, complications do occur.

**Electronic supplementary material** The online version of this chapter (doi:10.1007/978-3-319-19623-7_7) contains supplementary material, which is available to authorized users.

J.F. Kukleta
Hirslanden Klinik Im Park, Zurich, Switzerland
e-mail: jfkukleta@bluewin.ch

© Springer International Publishing Switzerland 2016
C. Avci, J.M. Schiappa (eds.), *Complications in Laparoscopic Surgery: A Guide to Prevention and Management*, DOI 10.1007/978-3-319-19623-7_7

Some complications arise from the patient's condition, but the most complications are avoidable. The systematic study of any possible or nearly impossible complications of any surgical procedure is the best way to understand its mechanism, to anticipate and to prevent it as far as possible. This is plan A on a checklist. Plan B is the list of solutions on how to manage the known complications. Plan C is the experience, the intuition and the knowledge of dealing with unexpected.

## 7.1    Introduction

Transabdominal preperitoneal hernia repair (TAPP) was first published by M. Arregui in 1992. The procedure consists of several phases. The first one is not hernia specific. Establishment of pneumoperitoneum, introduction of the endoscope, exploratory laparoscopy and confirmation of the preoperative diagnosis. Second phase is the preperitoneal dissection in a clearly defined area (landing zone) in order to retract all hernia sacs (with or without content) and any prolapsing fatty tissue and facilitate the following step (phase 3). Placement of a large ($15 \times 10$ cm or bigger) prosthetic mesh in the landing zone without any folds or wrinkles and taking measures to prevent early mesh dislocation (fixation, non-fixation). Phase 4 is the closure of the peritoneal opening and in phase 5 the $CO_2$ is evacuated and working port incisions are closed.

## 7.2    Classification of Complications

In order to diminish avoidable complications to absolute minimum, there must be a systematic workout of all possible deviations of a normal course. There is no general classification of complications in hernia repair that would allow direct comparison of the surgical techniques, because the differences may be very intervention specific. Important is of course not only the incidence of a complication but its severity too.

A general severity classification is e.g. the Clavien-Dindo classification, which was revised and validated in 2004, ranges from class I, denoting minimal deviation from the normal postoperative course without the need for pharmacological treatment or surgical, endoscopic or radiological intervention, to class V, indicating postoperative death.

Clavien-Dindo classification of postoperative complications:

I. Any deviation from the normal postoperative course without the need for pharmacological treatment or surgical, endoscopic and radiological interventions
II. Requiring pharmacological treatment with drugs other than such allowed for grade I complications
III. Requiring surgical, endoscopic or radiological intervention

IV. Life-threatening complication (including CNS complications) requiring IC/
    ICU management
V. Death of a patient

Despite the important value that this classification has, its use for TAPP repair of groin hernias is limited.

Thorough analysis of the whole procedure with all its obvious and hidden risks will be presented in order to help to prevent avoidable damage. It is difficult to avoid what is not well known. It is difficult to understand, if not well studied. It is easier to study the matter, if it is systematically described.

There is no generally accepted consensus on which deviation from "usual course" is or is not a complication. Therefore, the published results of complications may vary substantially.

Complications can be classified according to different aspects: according to consequences, to causality, to a specific phase of the procedure or the postoperative course.

## 7.2.1  In Relation to Consequences

| Minor | Haematoma, port-site infection, pneumonia, intestinal paralysis, early acute pain, urinary retention/ infection, seroma |
|-------|-------------------------------------------------------------------------------------------------------------------------|
| Major | Bladder injury, bowel injury, small bowel obstruction, big vessel injury, haemorrhage, mesh infection, trocar hernias, chronic pain, ischaemic orchitis and recurrence |

## 7.2.2  In Relation to Causality

Nonspecific
Related to e.g. general anaesthesia, OR table, burns
Laparoscopy
Access related, pneumoperitoneum related
Dissection technique
Vascular, nervous, organ injury, acute and chronic pain
Mesh
Infection, shrinkage, migration, recurrence, pain
Fixation
Acute and chronic pain, recurrence
Surgeon
Poor knowledge, poor orientation, poor performance

## 7.2.3  In Relation to Time

Intraoperative, early postoperative, late postoperative complications.

In his book "Chirurgie der Leistenhernie", Bittner et al. (2006) published the incidence of intraoperative, early postoperative and late postoperative complications on a large collective of patients undergoing a TAPP repair of *uncomplicated* primary unilateral and bilateral hernias.

## 7.2.4  Intraoperative Complications

| $n = 11{,}037$ | | |
|---|---|---|
| Bleeding (parietal, intra-abdominal) | 0.31 % | |
| Bladder injury | 0.0 % | (0.09 %) |
| Bowel injury | 0.0 % | (0.1 %) |
| Lesion of spermatic duct and vessels | 0.02 % | |
| Nerve injury (cutaneous femoral lateral) | 0.26 % | |
| Late (forced) conversion | 0.0 % | |
| Total | | (0.83 %) |

The numbers in brackets reflect all the hernia repairs performed including the complicated hernias too (recurrence, after preperitoneal repair open or laparoscopic, incarcerated or irreducible hernias, scrotal hernias and hernias after open prostatectomy or bladder surgery).

Some intraoperative complications may be specific for TAPP repair like visceral or bowel injuries, some may be addressed to general anaesthesia (circulatory complications, hypercarbia) and some result from incorrect dissection or misinterpretation of the local anatomy or too generous use of monopolar cautery.

## 7.2.5  Early Postoperative Complications

| $n = 11{,}037$ | |
|---|---|
| Urinary retention | 0.42 % |
| Haemorrhage | 0.26 % |
| Wound infection | 0.054 % |
| Mesh infection | 0.09 % |
| Small bowel obstruction | 0.036 % |
| Orchitis, epididymitis | 0.09 % |

## 7.2.6  Late Postoperative Complications

| $n = 11{,}037$ | | |
|---|---|---|
| Chronic pain | 0.045 % | |
| Seroma persistence, pseudohernia | 0.05 % | |
| Testicular atrophy | 0.05 % | |
| Ileus | 0.0 % | (0.03 %) |
| Recurrence | 0.69 % | |
| Trocar hernia | 0.56 % | |

The overall complication rate in this huge series is very low and reflects an immense experience of a dedicated team with a very high caseload (>1000/year). Under average conditions including teaching institutions, we have to assume that the true complication rate is much higher. The impact of experience as demonstrated by the same team shows how important is the standardisation of a new procedure, improving the operative skills, improving the anatomical knowledge and adhering strictly to the principals of minimal invasiveness in any TAPP hernia repair. In other reports from the early days of TAPP, one can recognise the same phenomenon of injuries to nervus cutaneus femoris lateralis due to imperfect knowledge of anatomy.

| Impact of experience | OP 1–600 | OP > 600 |
| --- | --- | --- |
| Nerve injury | 1.5 % | 0.19 % |
| Bleeding | 0.6 % | 0.23 % |
| Testicular atrophy | 0.3 % | 0.06 % |
| Recurrence rate | 4.8 % | 0.41 % |

## 7.3 Access-Related Complications (Phase 1)

To perform a TAPP repair, it needs the insufflation of 2–4 lt. of $CO_2$ to lift and expand the anterior abdominal wall to maintain the working space. This step carries a substantial risk of an injury to intra-abdominal structures.

Which is the safest and most effective method of establishing pneumoperitoneum and obtaining access to the abdominal cavity?

The safest and most efficient method of access is still controversial [1–4]. There are four ways on how to obtain access to the abdominal cavity:

(1) Open access (Hasson) (2) Veress needle to create pneumoperitoneum and trocar insertion without visual control (3) Direct trocar insertion (without previous pneumoperitoneum) (4) Visual entry with or without previous gas insufflation [7–12].

**IEHS Guidelines 2011** [13]
*Statements*
Level 1A    There is no definitive evidence that the open-entry technique for establishing pneumoperitoneum is superior or inferior to the other techniques currently available.
Level 1B    In thin patients (BMI < 27), the direct trocar insertion is a safe alternative to the Veress needle technique.
Level 2C    Establishing pneumoperitoneum to gain access to the abdominal cavity represents a potential risk of parietal, intra-abdominal and retroperitoneal injury. Patients after previous laparotomy, obese patients and very thin patients are at a higher risk.
Level 3    Waggling of the Veress needle from side to side must be avoided, because this can enlarge a 1.6-mm puncture injury to an injury of up to 1 cm in viscera or blood vessels.

Level 4       The various Veress needle safety tests or checks provide insufficient information on the placement of the Veress needle. The initial gas pressure when starting insufflation is a reliable indicator of correct intraperitoneal placement of the Veress needle. Left upper quadrant (LUQ, Palmer's) laparoscopic entry may be successful in patients with suspected or known periumbilical adhesions or history or presence of umbilical hernia or after three failed insufflation attempts at the umbilicus.

*Recommendations*

Grade A       When establishing pneumoperitoneum to gain access to the abdominal cavity, extreme caution is required. Be aware of the risk of injury. The open access should be utilised as an alternative to the Veress needle technique, especially in patients after previous open abdominal surgery.

## IEHS Update 2014 [14]

*New statements*—identical to previous except statement below.

Level 1B      In thin patients (BMI < 27), the direct trocar insertion is a safe alternative to the Veress needle technique (stronger evidence).

*New recommendations*—identical to previous except recommendation below.

Grade C       The direct trocar insertion (DTI) can be used in order to establish pneumoperitoneum as a safe alternative to Veress needle, Hasson approach or optical trocar, if patient's risk factors are considered and the surgeon is appropriately trained (new recommendation) [10].

Amongst general surgeons and gynaecologists, the most popular method is the Veress needle [1]. Although the open approach seems to be the safest, it does not eliminate the entire risk of injury [5, 6] (level 2C). When using open approach palpation through the peritoneal aperture, to exclude adhesions is mandatory before inserting a blunt cannula [6].

From Catarci et al. [5]

| N | | 12,919 patients |
|---|---|---|
| Method | Veress + 1st trocar | 82 % |
| | Hasson | 9 % |
| | Optical trocar | 9 % |
| Damage | Major vascular injury | 0.05 % |
| | Visceral lesions | 0.06 % |
| | Minor vascular injury | 0.07 % |
| | Overall morbidity | 0.18 % |
| Hasson | | 0.09 % |
| Veress + 1st trocar | | 0.18 % |
| Optical trocar | | 0.29 % |

## 7.4 Trocar-Related Complications

Further development of trocar design, from cutting instrument (to diminish the necessary penetrating force) towards the dilating instrument, has reduced the complication rate of parietal (or intra-abdominal) haemorrhage and the risk of developing a trocar hernia.

| Trocar parietal haemorrhage | |
| --- | --- |
| Cutting trocar | 1.76 % |
| Conical trocar | 0.056 % |
| | $p > 0.0001$ |
| Trocar hernia | |
| Cutting trocar | 1.27 % |
| Conical trocar | 0.037 % |
| | $p > 0.0001$ |

*Chirurgie der Leistenhernie*, Bittner et al., 2006

According to IEHS Guidelines and its Update, cutting trocars should not be used anymore. The use of 10 mm trocars or larger may predispose to hernias, especially in the umbilical region or in the oblique abdominal wall (stronger evidence) (level 2B). Therefore, fascial defects of 10 mm or bigger should be closed (stronger evidence) (grade B).

Concerning the closure of trocar wounds $\geq 10$ mm, I believe in closing the peritoneal layer too. The reason is the obvious difference in trocar hernia incidence in TAPP and TEP repair.

## 7.5 Dissection-Related Complications (Phase 2)

Poor knowledge of anatomy, not recognising the structures, wrong use of energy sources, impatience, lack of skills or too difficult dissection (e.g. after previous surgery) [16, 17] may lead to injury of big vessels, nerves, bowel, bladder, spermatic cord or spermatic vessels.

**Vessels "at risk"** Inferior epigastric, iliac and spermatic can be injured by the trocar, during the dissection or by fixing device.

**Nerves "at risk"(0.3 %)** During the dissection of the landing zone, the genital branch of the genitofemoral nerve, the lateral femoral cutaneous and the femoral nerve can be directly sectioned, damaged by coagulation or fixation device (see fixation-related complications below). The latter can injure even the ilioinguinal or iliohypogastric nerve depending on penetration depth of the device.

Major nerve injuries after laparoscopic hernioplasty have been reported, but the risk of this complication appears to be extremely low. In the early days of TAPP, these injuries reflected the lack of knowledge of the local anatomy or indelicate dissection.

The "triangle of pain" (lateral of spermatic vessels and below the iliopubic tract) as an area of nerves at risk had to be enlarged to about 1.5–2 cm above the iliopubic tract thanks to the brilliant anatomic study of Reinpold.

The incidence of sensory changes after a TAPP repair seems to be ten times lower than after an open repair ($p < 0.001$) [15].

## 7.6    Visceral Injuries (Bladder, Intestine) 0.1 %

**Keywords**  Veress needle, First and second trocar, Lack of overview, Delayed thermic lesions, Previous abdominal surgery, Lack of experience

Entering the abdominal cavity (with or without previous surgery) and during the preperitoneal dissection, there is an instant risk of bowel or bladder injury. Half of the big vessel injuries were reported to be caused by the second trocar! That means under visual control! Lack of force coordination or even worse lack of concentration may lead easily to a major complication. It is a great advantage of TAPP when compared to TEP that the procedure starts with existing working space. To move the long instruments in this space without endangering the fragile structures within is a must, but it is an ability developed after many laparoscopic operations. Even in easy repairs, the concentration must be maintained from the insertion of Veress needle till the last skin suture.

The chance to "look back" (from preperitoneal space to intraperitoneal space) during the dissection of the landing zone, especially in triangle of doom and triangle of pain, lets the operator control the bowel behind. Steeper Trendelenburg position may bring the bowel in safe distance.

Despite the fact that a urinary catheter is in general not recommended, in some complicated cases it may be of great value. Dissection after open prostatectomy or after previous prosthetic preperitoneal repair may become quite difficult. Not only the empty bladder, but the possibility of retrograde instillation (e.g. methylene blue) may be advantageous to detect and control eventual bladder injury.

In case of necessary adhesiolysis, any suspicion of serosal lesion must be scrutinised. Oversewn serosa tear is more secure than a missed one.

The adhesiolysis of hernia content is not advisable. The hernia sac (e.g. in sliding hernias) is mobilised in toto with the content during the preperitoneal dissection.

The most dangerous condition is the unrecognised enterotomy or delayed enterotomy. The latter mostly caused by inappropriate use of monopolar cautery with consecutive tissue necrosis and delayed onset of postoperative peritonitis. Therefore, even after an easy procedure, stay alert to any unusual symptom after a laparoscopic hernia repair.

## 7.7    Seroma, Haematoma 0.29–4 %

**Keywords**  Pseudo-recurrence, Hernia size, Hernia type, Rare reoperation 0.46 %, Aspiration seldom necessary [20].

The bigger the hernia sac is, the bigger the chance of development of a seroma formation.

In large indirect sacs, the recommended complete retraction may lead to higher incidence of haematomas and may compromise the blood supply to the testicle. The transection of the indirect sac and leaving the distal portion open shows higher incidence of seromas and may lead in later course to development of a pseudo-hydrocoele. Fixing the distal portion to the abdominal wall lateral to epigastric vessels seems to help to avoid the occurrence of seromas [26].

In larger direct hernias (M2-3), the incidence of seromas can be significantly reduced by inversion of transversalis fascia and fixation to Cooper's ligament with tacks [18, 19] or using an Endoloop [24, 25]. This step diminishes the dead space for seroma formation but additionally obliterates the potential of mesh dislocation into previous hernia space.

Inversion of the transversalis fascia is associated with a statistically lower incidence of postoperative seroma, without increasing postoperative pain despite the use of one or two additional tacks [19].

**Update IEHS**
*New statements*—identical to previous except statement below.
Level 4    Alternatively to fixation of the extended fascia transversalis to Copper's ligament, the direct inguinal hernia defect can be closed by a pre-tied suture loop. (new statement).
*New recommendations*—identical to previous except recommendation below.
Grade D    As an alternative, the primary closure of direct inguinal hernia defects with a pre-tied suture loop can be used (new recommendation).

**New Literature [24]**
Prospective study, 250 patients, , 94 direct hernias, 76 were M2 or M3, were treated with ligation of the everted direct sac with PDS Endoloop [24]. 1.3 % residual seroma at 3 months, no chronic groin pain and no hernia recurrence after a median follow-up of 18 months.

Conclusion: The primary closure of direct inguinal hernia defects with a pre-tied suture loop during endoscopic TEP repair is safe, efficient and very reliable for the prevention of postoperative seroma formation, without increasing the risk of developing chronic groin pain or hernia recurrence.

## 7.8    Urinary Retention: POUR 0.42–3.1 %

POUR is probably of multifactorial origin. There is no general indication for preoperative catheterisation, and there are no clear predictive factors for postoperative retention. It is advisable that the patient empties the bladder before surgery. Full urinary bladder during a TAPP repair increases the risk of a bladder injury and can make the dissection even more difficult. In patients with expected technical difficulties (after previous abdominal, prostatic or bladder surgery) or extended operating time (bilateral scrotal, in learning curve), preoperative catheterisation should be considered.

Postoperative urinary retention is more frequent in endoscopic repairs (under general anaesthesia – GA) then in open hernia repairs under local anaestesia, possibly due to inhibitory effect of GA on bladder function [27].

Urinary retention may significantly prolong the hospital stay. With consequent approach towards possible POUR—preoperative emptying, restrictive fluid management in the early postoperative phase, early mobilisation and refrain from opioids—the incidence of retention can be as low as 0.5 % [28].

## 7.9    Testicular Problems 0.15 %

### 7.9.1    Testicular Atrophy (0.04–0.09 %)

**Keywords** Testicular pain, Hydrocoele, Ischemic orchitis, Venous congestion, Nerve irritations, Leaving the indirect sack in situ

### 7.9.2    How to Avoid Testicular Problems?

The early postoperative tenderness of testis is often related to dissectional trauma or just irritation of genital branch of the genitofemoral nerve. Gentle dissection in correct plane with preservation of spermatic fascia protects the nerve; prudent use of monopolar cautery is most probably safer than incomplete haemostasis. Separating peritoneum from spermatic cord and vessels (parietalisation) seems to be easier if these structures were lifted by the nondominant instrument and the peritoneum pulled down by the dominant instrument. However, this is absolutely not necessary; there is always a way to grasp adjacent tissue to facilitate this step and avoid any possible injury to spermatic structures. The "no touch technique" is our policy.

Another possible reason for testicular pain was the lateral slit in mesh in order to pass the lower tail under the cord and vessels and close it again with the upper tail (analog Lichtenstein). The idea of slitting the mesh was to prevent the dislocation of the low lateral corner above the triangle of pain. The solution to this is a generous parietalisation and a non-penetrating fixation with fibrin sealant or cyanoacrylate glue. Late transection of spermatic duct caused by shrinkage of a slit mesh was published. The IEHS Guidelines do not recommend slitting the mesh (see below).

## 7.10    Mesh-Related Complications

### 7.10.1 Mesh Shrinkage

#### 7.10.1.1 Factor Mesh Material vs. Mesh Construction
Not only variable polymers (polypropylene PP, polyester PE, polytetrafluoroethylene PTFE or polyvinylidene fluoride PVDF) but the mesh product itself induces

different behaviour of the recipient after the mesh is implanted. Mesh size, its strength, total foreign body weight, porosity (the most important property), shrinkage rate, bridging and flexural rigidity may influence the final outcome.

The microporous meshes (most often heavyweight meshes) show an excessive shrinkage rate (compression by the scar tissue formation as a consequence of a strong inflammatory foreign body reaction). The most modern mesh products are macroporous. The difference between the macroporous lightweight meshes and the microporous heavyweight meshes in form of less local discomfort, chronic pain or a foreign body feeling could not be demonstrated in any study of TAPP or TEP repair.

## 7.10.2 Mesh Infections

Mesh infections in TAPP are nearly inexistent, but anecdotic reports were published [29–32].

## 7.10.3 Recurrence TAPP 0.27–3.7 %

### 7.10.3.1 Reasons for Recurrence

**Technique**
Lack of experience
Insufficient extent of dissection
Missed hernia
Preperitoneal lipoma
Suboptimal mesh placement
Inappropriate retention/fixation
Mesh lifted by haematoma
Inferior lateral mesh edge lifted at closure

**Material**
Microporous mesh
Heavyweight mesh/excessive shrinkage
Size to small
Insufficient overlap in relation to shrinkage
Mesh slit
Mesh protrusion

**Risk Factors**
Collagen disease
Smoking
Obesity
Malnutrition
Diabetes Type ll

Chronic lung disease
Coagulopathy
Steroids
Radiotherapy, chemotherapy
Jaundice
Male gender
Anaemia

The most important causes of recurrence after a TAPP repair are avoidable. Small mesh, insufficient extent of dissection, incorrect mesh placement, slotted mesh, missed lipoma, sliding retroperitoneal fat, insufficient fixation, non-fixation in a wrong indication, all of them being a technical underestimation of a true problem rather than lack of knowledge [31, 36].

The recommended mesh size for TAPP repair is $15 \times 10$ cm or larger [14, 33–35]. Smaller meshes are the most important cause of hernia recurrence today.

Mesh slit should have had prevented possible mesh dislocation, instead of that it increased the recurrence rate [33]. Leibl demonstrates that both small mesh size and the slit in mesh increased the risk for recurrence. Heikinnen [38] changes his policy in TAPP repair from Surgipro $6 \times 10$ cm to Prolene $10 \times 14$ cm and reduces his recurrence rate from 28 to 0 %. Felix [37] found in six patients with chronic testicular pain four patients with a keyholed mesh. It might be speculated whether the slit predisposed the nerve to injury or chronic irritation from the mesh.

| Phase 1 | Slitted mesh, $13 \times 8$ cm |
| --- | --- |
| Cause of recurrence | Mesh too small |
| Recurrence rate | 2.8 % slit region insufficient |
| Phase 2 | Nonslotted, $15 \times 10$ cm |
| Cause of recurrence | Mesh dislocation |
| Recurrence rate | 0.36 % |

From Leibl et al. [33]

## 7.10.4 Pseudo-recurrence

Seroma in the early postoperative course maybe wrongly understood as a recurrence. Ultrasound helps to clarify. Overlooked lipoma in inguinal or femoral canal may present as a recurrence too and will most probably lead to a revision or removal through anterior approach after the nature of the local swelling was confirmed by MRI.

Protrusion of a lightweight mesh into a large direct defect is rare, but a true recurrence, despite the correct size and placement of the prosthetic material. In such situation, meshes with higher flexural rigidity are recommended.

### 7.10.5  Mesh Displacement, Erosion, Migration

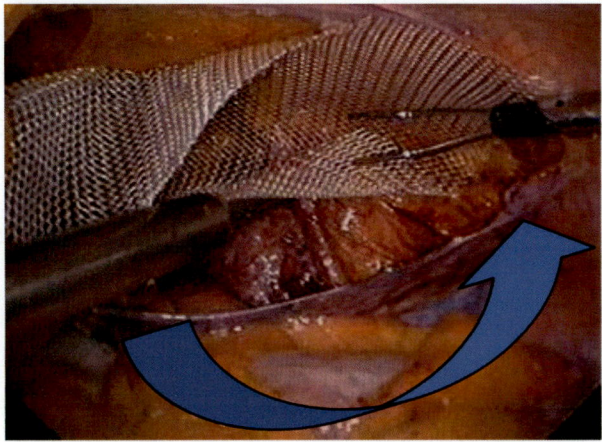

The most common reason for a mesh dislocation is its insufficient size and imperfect placement. The lower margin of the "landing zone" has to allow placing the mesh over psoas muscle without lifting up the low lateral mesh corner when closing the peritoneum. Penetrating fixation (staples, tackers, sutures, etc.) do not compensate for "incorrect" placement. Soft fixation (sealants and glues) may prevent an early movement and decrease the recurrence rate.

Excessive shrinkage of some meshes may also contribute to mesh displacement or to "meshoma" formation.

The few but true reports of late migration and erosion into adjacent organs stress again the importance of strict adherence to the rules of TAPP repair. These unusual complications seem to be the consequence of technical errors [39–46].

### 7.11    Fixation-Related Complications

#### 7.11.1  Haemorrhage, Injury to Nerves, Acute Pain, Chronic Pain, Recurrence

Knowledge of the local anatomy should eliminate the risk of injury of big- and medium-sized vessels during dissection or mesh fixation. Penetrating fixation seemed in the past to be necessary to prevent mesh dislocation. Over time, we have learned that mesh retention rather than fixation is only a temporary need, until host tissue ingrowth will take place. The macroporosity of the implant would support the ingrowth without pronounced shrinkage. This fact led to the introduction of fibrin sealant and glue fixation [76–80, 83–86].

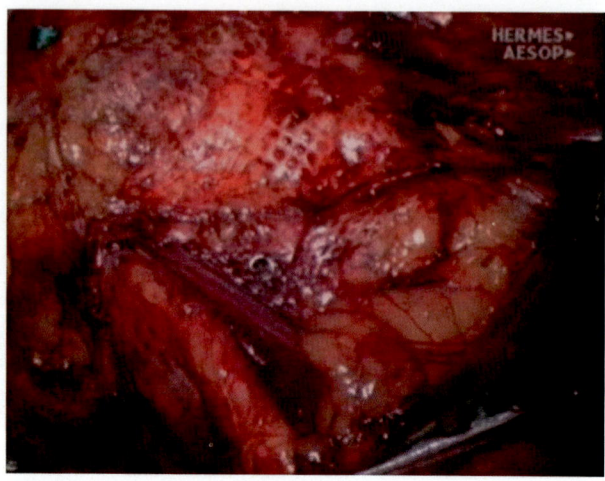

A spiral tack injuring genitofemoral nerve (Courtesy of Jorge Cervantes, Mexico)

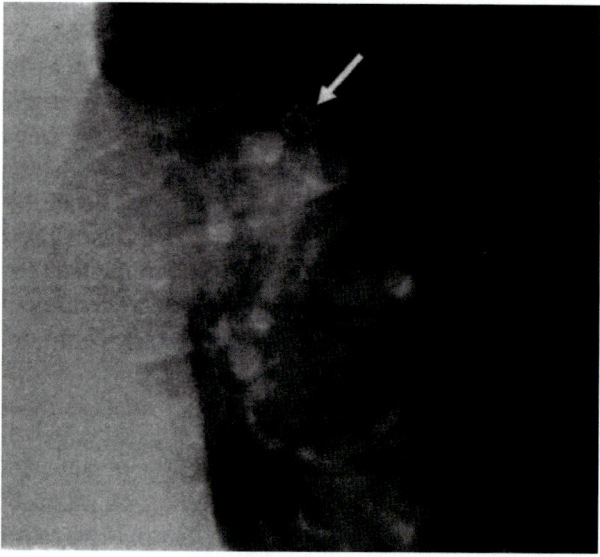

Tack in pulmonary artery after TEP (Courtesy of Jorge Cervantes, Mexico)

Penetrating fixation does not compensate if the mesh is too small. Temptation to fix the mesh with tackers, staples or sutures in triangle of doom or triangle of pain can lead to disasters. For example, in order to prevent the dislocation of "the critical corner" causing a long-lasting neuropathy of genitofemoral nerve.

There is a clear trend in TAPP and TEP repair towards soft fixation or non-fixation [47–52].

Lovisetto [53] compared in a RCT staples vs. fibrin glue mesh fixation in TAPP repair. It shows a lower incidence of postoperative neuralgia and an earlier resumption of physical and social activities in patients with soft fixation.

Kapiris [22] publishes excellent recurrence rate of 0.16 % in a large cohort of TAPP repairs with 15×10 cm meshes and no fixation in a long follow-up.

Akolekar [54] shows a rise of recurrence rate in TEP repair with non-fixed meshes since the introduction of lightweight meshes. All above teams are experts in their discipline, so the simple technical errors are less probable.

There is probably more than just the mesh size and its rigidity. The size of the defect both in direct as well as indirect hernias shows even in open repairs the higher risk for recurrence.

## 7.12 Conversion 0.0–6.2 %

Conversions in TAPP are very rare. Hostile abdomen should be ruled out preoperatively as a relative contraindication for TAPP due to inadequate risk of bowel injury. However, even after uncomplicated appendectomy, cholecystectomy or C-section, one can encounter extensive omento-parietal adhesions. Depending on surgeon's experience and the extent of adhesions, it is wise to convert early enough before damage is done. Unforced conversion to open anterior repair can lead to better results; forced conversion as an "ultima ratio" after serious injury lead to laparotomy and higher complications rate. Lack of overview can lead to missed enterotomy with all its consequences.

Prudent patient selection, proper teaching and enough self-criticism are the best counsellors.

## 7.13 Closure-Related Complications

### 7.13.1 Small Bowel Obstruction

**IEHS Guidelines on Peritoneal Closure**
*Statements*

Level 3    Incomplete peritoneal closure or its breakdown in endoscopic, preperitoneal hernia repair increases the risk of bowel obstruction.

Level 3    TAPP procedure presents a higher statistical risk of small bowel obstruction than TEP.

Level 5    The most appropriate peritoneal closure is achieved by running absorbable suture.

Level 5    Running suture seems to cause less pain compared with clip/tack closure.

Level 5    The closure of entrance of indirect sacs may reduce the risk of internal hernia with consecutive incarceration, strangulation or small bowel obstruction.

*Recommendations*

Grade C    A thorough closure of peritoneal incision or peritoneal tears should be done.

Grade D    The peritoneal closure can be accomplished by a running suture.

Bowel obstruction can develop due to adhesions between omentum or epiploic appendices and suture line, between the mesh and the intestines, e.g. caused by inadequate closure of a peritoneal lesion [55–57]. The peritoneal opening must be thoroughly closed to prevent contact of viscera with the prosthetic mesh material and to reduce the risk of bowel obstruction. This closure can be achieved with staples, tackers, running suture or glue. These last two methods are more time-consuming but less painful [58, 59] (see Chap. 9). Rare cases of bowel obstruction in port-site hernias also have been described, especially after TAPP. Several anecdotic reports on small bowel obstruction both in TAPP [60] and TEP repairs have been published [61, 62]. The data from Swedish National Inguinal Hernia Register show higher incidence of late postoperative bowel obstruction after TAPP than after TEP [55].

### IEHS Guidelines Update on Peritoneal Closure

*New statements*—identical to previous.

*New recommendations*—identical to previous except the statement below.

Grade B    A thorough closure of peritoneal incision or of bigger peritoneal tears should be achieved (stronger evidence).

The previous recommendation on peritoneal closure already connoted verbally the importance of the task, although assigned to Grade C. To emphasise the fact, this recommendation was upgraded to Grade B.

Ross et al. [63] reported that the postoperative activity limitation at 2 weeks was significantly better in the suture group when compared to the stapled group ($p=0.005$). Additionally, sutured PF closure had less early postoperative pain when compared to the tacker group ($p=0.038$). He concluded: Following TAPP IHR, suture closure of the peritoneal flaps significantly improve 2-week postoperative movement limitation compared to stapled and tacked peritoneal closure.

Köhler et al. [64] raise attention to a new cause of small bowel obstruction owing to strained adhesions and ingrowth between a small bowel segment and a polyglyconate unidirectional self-anchoring barbed suture device (V-lock) (this has to be cut short at the end of a running suture).

Similar report was presented by Fitzgerald et al. [65]—small bowel obstruction due to displaced spiral tack.

### 7.13.2  Port-Site Hernias 0–6.2 %

Port-site hernia is a late postoperative complication predominantly reported in TAPP repair. Although, according to general opinion, only 10 mm and bigger trocar site defects should be closed [14, 35, 66], development of incisional hernia with consequences was described even with 3–5 mm trocars [67, 68].

**IEHS Guidelines Update 2014 raises the questions: What kind of trocars should be used? Is there any relation between the trocar type and risk of injury and/or trocar hernias?**

*New statement*—identical to previous except statement below.

Level 2B    The use of 10-mm trocars or larger may predispose to hernias, especially in the umbilical region or in the oblique abdominal wall (stronger evidence).

*New recommendation*—identical to previous except recommendation below.

Grade B    Fascial defects of 10 mm or bigger should be closed (stronger evidence). Upgraded.

The design of dilating, instead of cutting trocars, contributed significantly to decrease the risk of port-site bleeding and development of port-site hernias [59, 69–72]. Bittner et al. found significant differences in incidence of trocar-related parietal haemorrhage (cutting trocar 1.76 vs. 0.056 % conical trocar, $p > 0.0001$) and incidence of trocar hernias (cutting trocar 1.27 vs. 0.037 % conical trocar, $p > 0.0001$)

## 7.14    Chronic Pain 0.03–2.2 %

The aetiology of chronic pain (CP) is still not exactly known; it seems to be of multifactorial origin (surgeon-related, mesh-related and patient-related causes). It is often associated with incorrect dissection, with inadequate use of monopolar cautery; with penetrating and/or permanent fixation, with anatomically incorrect fixation, with patient's individual inflammatory response to local dissection, with the implant or with pre-existent pain syndrome. Chronic postoperative pain following TAPP and TEP is more prevalent than recurrence [73]. Preoperative pain, repair for recurrent groin hernias (following anterior repair) and younger age at surgery seem to predict development of chronic postoperative pain. Identification of "patients at risk" may improve the choice of surgical procedure and reduce morbidity and cost [74, 75].

The randomised study by Singh et al. [81] showed that preoperative pain, younger age, open surgery and 7-day postoperative pain were independent risk factors for chronic pain.

Chronic pain syndrome is seldom seen in endoscopic hernia repair [82]. According to Aasvang et al. [83], the overall incidence of chronic pain after open groin hernia repair is 18 % (range, 0–75.5 %) and 6 % after endoscopic repair (range, 1–16 %; $p=0.01$)

The risk of acute and chronic pain is lower after endoscopic groin hernia repair compared with open surgery with or without mesh. The risk of sensory disturbances of the groin is lower after endoscopic groin hernia repair compared with open surgery with or without mesh [79].

No consensus guidelines exist for the management of postoperative chronic pain yet [73, 76], despite many scientific papers about this troublesome condition during the last 10 years. There is a need for guidelines regarding management of chronic pain.

In between, it is more important to try to avoid anything that could lead to CP. Anatomically correct and gentle dissection, wise use of cautery, macroporous meshes, noninvasive fixation using glues or sealants or no fixation in P, L1-2/ M1-2 hernias, no tackers when closing peritoneum, correct indication for surgery and proper choice of patients, considering their individual factors seem to be the right way to go.

## 7.15 Infertility, Dysejaculation?

Although animal studies have suggested a strong correlation between mesh inguinal hernia repairs and structural damage to elements of the spermatic cord and testicle [89], this has not translated into a clinically significant infertility rate after open or laparoscopic inguinal hernia repair [14] (Fitzgibbons in Update of IEHS Guidelines), [87, 88].

*New Statement*
Level 2B    Inguinal hernia repair with mesh is not associated with an increased risk of, or clinically important risk for, male infertility.

*New Recommendation*
Grade B    Groin hernia repair using mesh techniques may continue to be performed without major concern about the risk for male infertility.

Peeters [90] reported a possible adverse effect on sperm motility 1 year after TEP repair with lightweight meshes, but could not confirm it at 3 years follow-up [91].

In a Danish study including men undergoing laparoscopic inguinal hernia repair who were registered in the Danish Hernia Database, dysejaculation occurred in 3.1 % [92].

## 7.16 Management of Possible Problems

### 7.16.1 Pneumoperitoneum

If using Veress needle, lift the skin with two graspers/forceps. After 3 nonsuccessful punctures periumbilically, use another localisation (Palmer's point, subcostal left) or open access (Hasson). When the abdomen does not grow despite of proper gas flow, think of having punctured a hollow organ (stomach, bladder, intestine). Search for a possible injury, after introducing the endoscope, at the place where you punctured (posterior wall, vessels).

### 7.16.2 Trocar Injury

Immediate resolution recommended.

*Serosa lesions* of bowel loop: it is, probably, preferable to suture after placement of working ports.

*Small bowel full-thickness lesion* without massive spillage—intra-abdominal suture is possible. In doubt, do not expect typical fluid coming out of the lesion because of the intra-abdominal pressure. If not enough skilled, exteriorise the loop and repair outside. In case of no gross contamination, cover with omentum major and proceed with the rest of surgery.

*Large bowel lesions* must be thoroughly sutured. In case of obvious contamination, the surgeon shall proceed to a change of strategy: either open repair or postpone mesh implantation until one is sure the suture was successful and there's no active peritonitis going on.

*Parietal bleeding*: Haemostasis with compression, peanuts soaked with diluted adrenalin, bipolar coagulation or suture. Control the result at reduced IAP. Remember that cutting trocars belong to museum.

*Injury of big vessels*: laparotomy.

*Conversion*: preferably unforced decision before too late. Repair what you can repair; otherwise call for a specialist.

### 7.16.3 Dissectional Injuries

In all patients, especially in those under any kind of anticoagulation (even Aspirin cardio) or with coagulopathy, consequent haemostasis is required. Do not rely on nature or drains.

*Epigastric vessels*: Prefer clips rather than just coagulation, transfascial sutures below and above the lesion. The closer to the iliac vessels, the more difficult it may get to repair the damage.

*Iliac vessels*: Be aware of the anatomy; stay away, at respectful controllable distance. Behave as requested in triangle of doom and in triangle of pain.

*Corona mortis, suprapubic vessels, vessels around the femoral canal*: These vessels have to be left where they are. Remember anatomy. Keeping the operative field dry guarantees better orientation and recognition of the important structures.

*Bladder injury*: If in doubt, retrograde instillation of diluted methylene blue, suture and Foley catheter. In case of previous surgery in preperitoneal space (TAPP, TEP, prostatectomy, section alta, etc.), anticipate problems and catheterise preoperatively.

### 7.16.4 Postoperative Problems

*Acute postoperative pain*: Most patients have after TAPP repair very moderate or even low level of pain in the first 12 h. Unexpected and inadequate acute pain asks for explanation. Early re-laparoscopy rules out doubts; explant tackers or staples if used.

*Peritonitis*: Early revision laparoscopy recommended.

*Ileus*: Early re-laparoscopy

*Infection*: Drainage, antibiotics, mesh removal

*Seroma*: Inform patients preoperatively, wait, aspirate after 1–3 months and operate after 6–12 months if still symptomatic.

*Chronic pain*: Wait, take care of pain, accompany the patient; most get better and will not need any treatment in the future. Contact a local pain centre; rule out other possible pain causes. Concern involving specialists, local and peripheral infiltrations. Do not try to reoperate before 6–12 months, unless you have found a clear reason to do so.

*Recurrence*: In case of a rare recurrence after a TAPP repair, use the opposite (open) approach if not already has been used previously (recurrence after Lichtenstein/mesh-free tissue repair and TAPP/TEP). Try to find out the true reason for recurrence (e.g. small mesh, no fixation, lightweight mesh in a big direct hernia) and consider your experience before you decide to proceed.

### 7.16.5 How to Prevent Complications?

Even the most simple primary groin hernia deserves full attention. Profound knowledge of anatomy of both anterior and posterior approach to groin hernia repair is indispensable. Consequent haemostasis is the key. Good overview and correct anatomical orientation prevent the majority of possible complications.

"TAPP repair" is a very well-standardised procedure. Although the average operation time is a kind of a mirror of operator's experience, the surgery takes as long as it is necessary to accomplish the so-called perfect repair. Indirect hernia, e.g. takes longer than the direct one. Do not forget what the objective of a hernia repair is: Patient's satisfaction!

It is the surgeon's state of mind that creates higher demands in order to achieve the best possible results.

Obey the rules: pneumoperitoneum, dilating trocar, under direct vision, consequent haemostasis, cautious use of cautery, cautious adhesiolysis, convert before too late, stay away of big vessels, respect nerves. Noninvasive fixation if any, adequate mesh size. Complete closure of peritoneal gap and closure of trocar incision (Table 7.1).

## 7.17 Summary

The overall complication rate in laparo-endoscopic hernia repair is low. True incidence of complications is in fact unknown, because of underreporting. The individual surgeon determines the outcome far more than the procedure he chooses to use.

Complications are avoidable by awareness, knowledge, proper teaching and mentoring, disciplined dissection, perfection of skills, attention to details, wise selection of patients and experience.

How to avoid a complication?

Prevent it!

How to prevent a complication?

Follow the correct path, anticipate possible complications and act accordingly (start re-reading the above thoughts).

**Table 7.1** Reports of complications after laparoscopic hernia repair

| Author | Operation | Intestinal obstruction | Lipogranuloma | Haematoma | Other |
|---|---|---|---|---|---|
| Sailors | R: TAPP48 | 1 | 2 | 2-scrotal ecchymosis: 4-groin swelling; 2-testicular asymmetry | |
| Wegener | TAPP | 1 | | | |
| Paget | R: TAPP 222 | | | 6-seroma: 5-urinary retention: 1-hydrocoele; 1-small bowel perf | |
| Angelescu | R: TAPP 50 | | 1 | 2-seroma; 1-mesh migration | |
| Azurin | TEP | 1 | | | |
| Havlik | P: TEP 20 | | 1 | 1-OP | |
| Klopfenstein | TEP | | | | 1-SE |
| Schurz | R: NS 156 | | 3 | 4-TP; 1-A; 1-UD | |
| Giuly | TAPP | | | | 1-OP |
| Baladas | TAPP | 1 | | | |
| Rodda | | 1 | | | |
| Eugene | TEP | 1 | | | |
| Goodwin | TAPP | | | | 1-AS in PS |
| Pennekamp | | | | Retroperitoneal | |
| Kazantsev | NS | | | | 1-ECF |
| Ridings | R: TAPP 1700 | 3 | | 1-visceral injury | |
| Michel | TAPP | | | | 1-PG |
| Mincheff | TEP | | | | 1-FTI |
| Rieger | TAPP | | | | 1-CVF |
| Lau | TEP | | | | 1-PC |

From Singh-Ranger et al. [32]
*NS* not stated, *SE* subcutaneous emphysema, *PS* port site, *OP* osteitis pubis, *PC* preperitoneal collection, *FTI* focal testicular infarction, *CVF* colovesical fistula, *ECF* enterocutaneous fistula, *AS* appendicular strangulation, *PG* pyoderma gangrenosum, *UD* undefined, *A* abdominal, *TP* transperitoneal, *R* retrospective study, *P* prospective study

# References

1. Vilos GA, Vilos AG, Abu-Rafea B, Hollett-Caines J, Nikkhah-Abyaneh Z, Edris F (2009) Three simple steps during closed laparoscopic entry may minimize major injuries. Surg Endosc 23(4):758–764
2. Shamiyeh A, Glaser K, Kratochwill H, Hörmandinger K, Fellner F, Wayand W, Zehetner J (2009) Lifting of the umbilicus for the installation of pneumoperitoneum with the Veress needle increases the distance to the retroperitoneal and intraperitoneal structures. Surg Endosc 23:313–317, 3

3. Vilos GA, Ternamian A, Dempster J, Laberge PY, The Society of Obstetricians and gynaecologists of Canada (2007) Laparoscopic entry: a review of techniques, technologies, and complications. J Obstet Gynaecol Can 29:433–465, 1A

4. Teoh B, Sen R, Abbot J (2005) An evaluation of four tests used to ascertain Verres needle placement at closed laparoscopy. J Minim Invasive Gynecol 12(4):153–158

5. Catarci M, Carlini M, Gentileschi P, Santoro E (2001) Major and minor injuries during the creation of pneumoperitoneum: a multicenter study on 12,919 cases. Surg Endosc 15:566–569 (2C)

6. Hasson HM (1971) A modified instrument and method for laparoscopy. Am J Obstet Gynecol 110:886–887 (5)

7. Peitgen K, Nimtz K, Hellinger A, Walz MK (1997) Open approach or Veress needle in laparoscopic interventions? Results of a prospective randomized controlled study [in German]. Chirurg 68:910–913 (2B)

8. Neudecker J, Sauerland S, Neugebauer E, Bergamaschi R, Bonjer HJ, Cuschieri A, Fuchs KH, Jacobi C, Janson FW, Koivusalo AM, Lacy A, McMahon MJ, Millat B, Schwenk W (2002) The EAES clinical practice guideline on the pneumoperitoneum for laparoscopic surgery. Surg Endosc 16:1121–1143 (2C)

9. Merlin TL, Hiller JE, Maddern GJ, Jamieson GG, Brown AR, Kolbe A (2003) Systematic review of the safety and effectiveness of methods used to establish pneumoperitoneum in laparoscopic surgery. Br J Surg 90:668–679 (1A)

10. Agresta F, De Simone P, Ciardo LF, Bedin N (2004) Direct trocar insertion vs Veress needle in nonobese patients undergoing laparoscopic procedures: a randomized prospective single-center study. Surg Endosc 18:1778–1781 (1B)

11. Altun H, Banli O, Kavlakoglu B, Ku¨cu¨kkayikci B, Kelesoglu C, Erez N (2007) Comparison between direct trocar and Veress needle insertion in laparoscopic cholecystectomy. J Laparoendosc Adv Surg Tech A 17:709–712 (1B)

12. Orlando R, Palatini P, Lirussi F (2003) Needle and trocar injuries in diagnostic laparoscopy under local anesthesia: what is the true incidence of these complications? J Laparoendosc Adv Surg Tech A 13(3):181–184

13. Bittner R, Arregui ME, Bisgaard T, Dudai M, Ferzli GS, Fitzgibbons RJ, Fortelny RH, Klinge U, Kockerling F, Kuhry E, Kukleta J, Lomanto D, Misra MC, Montgomery A, Morales-Conde S, Reinpold W, Rosenberg J, Sauerland S, Schug-Pass C, Singh K, Timoney M, Weyhe D, Chowbey P (2011) Guidelines for laparoscopic (TAPP) and endoscopic (TEP) treatment of inguinal hernia [International Endohernia Society (IEHS)]. Surg Endosc 25:2773–2843 (1A)

14. Bittner R, Arregui ME, Bisgaard T, Dudai M, Ferzli GS, Fitzgibbons RJ, Fortelny RH, Klinge U, Kockerling F, Kuhry E, Kukleta J, Lomanto D, Misra MC, Montgomery A, Morales-Conde S, Reinpold W, Rosenberg J, Sauerland S, Schug-Pass C, Singh K, Timoney M, Weyhe D, Chowbey P (2014) Update of guidelines on laparoscopic (TAPP) and endoscopic (TEP) treatment of inguinal hernia (International Endohernia Society) (IEHS). Surg Endosc. doi:10.1007/s00464-011-1799-6

15. Gillion JF, Fagniez PL (1999) Chronic pain and cutaneous sensory changes after inguinal hernia repair: comparison between open and laparoscopic techniques. Hernia 3:75–80.

16. MacFadyen BV Jr, Arregui ME, Corbitt JD, Filipi CJ, Fitzgibbons RJ Jr, Franklin ME, McKernan JB, Olsen DO, Phillips EH, Rosenthal D, Schultz LS, Sewell RW, Smoot RT, Spaw AT, Toy FK, Waddell RL, Zucker KA (1993) Complications of laparoscopic herniorrhaphy. Surg Endosc 7:155–158

17. Phillips EH, Arregui M, Carroll BJ, Corbitt J, Crafton WB, Fallas MJ, Filipi R, Fitzgibbons RJ, Franklin MJ, McKernan B, Olsen D, Ortega A, Payne JH Jr, Peters J, Rodriguez R, Rosette P, Schultz L, Seld A, Sewell R, Smoot R, Toy F, Waddell R, Watson S (1995) Incidence of complications following laparoscopic hernioplasty. Surg Endosc 9:16–21

18. Jehaes C (1995) Laparoscopic extraperitoneal approach for inguinal hernia repair in Inguinal hernia repair. In: Schumpelick V, Wantz GE (eds) Inguinal hernia repair. Karger, Basel, pp 269–2722

19. Reddy VM, Sutton CD, Bloxham L, Garcea G, Ubhi SS, Robertson GS (2007) Laparoscopic repair of direct inguinal hernia: a new technique that reduces the development of postoperative seroma. Hernia 11:393–396. doi:10.1007/s10029-007-0233-4

20. Lau H, Lee F (2003) Seroma following endoscopic extraperitoneal inguinal hernioplasty. Surg Endosc 17(11):1773–1777, Epub 2003 Jun 17. Prospective study, 450 patients, 533 TEPs, primary objective incidence and treatment of seromas after TEPP

21. Litwin DE, Pham QN, Oleniuk FH, Kluftinger AM, Rossi L (1997) Laparoscopic groin hernia surgery: the TAPP procedure. Transabdominal preperitoneal hernia repair. Can J Surg 40:192–198

22. Kapiris A, Brough WA, Royston CM, O'Boyle C, Sedman PC (2001) Laparoscopic transabdominal preperitoneal (TAPP) hernia repair. A 7-year two-center experience in 3017 patients. Surg Endosc 15:972–975

23. Cihan A, Ozdemir H, Uçan BH, Acun Z, Comert M, Tascilar O, Cesur A, Cakmak GK, Gundogdu S (2006) Fade or fate. Seroma in laparoscopic inguinal hernia repair. Surg Endosc 20(2):325–328, Epub 2005 Dec 5

24. Berney CR (2012) The Endoloop technique for the primary closure of direct inguinal hernia defect during the endoscopic totally extraperitoneal approach. Hernia 16(3):301–305. doi:10.1007/s10029-011-0892-z, Epub 2011 Nov 27

25. Köckerling F, Jacob DA, Lomanto D, Chowbey P, Berney CR (2012) The Endoloop technique for the primary closure of direct inguinal hernia defect during the endoscopic totally extraperitoneal approach. Hernia 16(4):493–494. doi:10.1007/s10029-012-0920-7

26. Daes J (2014) Endoscopic repair of large inguinoscrotal hernias: management of the distal sac to avoid seroma formation. Hernia 18:119–122. doi:10.1007/s10029-012-1030-2

27. Jensen P, Mikkelsen T, Kehlet H (2002) Postherniorrhaphy urinary retention—effect of local, regional, and general anesthesia: a review. Reg Anesth Pain Med 27:612–617

28. Bittner R, Schmedt CG, Schwarz J, Kraft K, Leibl BJ (2002) Laparoscopic transperitoneal procedure for routine repair of groin hernia. Br J Surg 89:1062–1066

29. Hofbauer C, Andersen PV, Juul P, Qvist N (1998) Late mesh rejection as a complication to transabdominal preperitoneal laparoscopic hernia repair. Surg Endosc 12:1164–1165

30. Michel P, Wullstein C, Hopt UT (2001) Pyoderma gangrenosum after TAPP hernioplasty. A rare necrotizing wound infection differential diagnosis. Chirurg 72:1501–1503

31. Bittner R, Leibl B, Kraft K, Daübler P, Schwarz J (1996) Laparoscopic herniorrhaphy (TAPP)—complications and recurrences following 900 operations. Zentralbl Chir 121:313–319

32. Singh-Ranger D, Taneja T, Sroden P, Peters J (2007) A rare complication following laparoscopic TEP repair: case report and discussion of the literature. Hernia 11:453–456

33. Leibl B et al (2000) Recurrence after endoscopic transperitoneal hernia repair (TAPP): causes, reparative techniques, and results of the reoperation. J Am Coll Surg 190:651–655

34. Eklund A, Rudberg C, Leijonmarck CE, Rasmussen I, Spangen L, Wickbom G, Wingren U, Montgomery A (2007) Recurrent inguinal hernia: randomized multicenter trial comparing laparoscopic and Lichtenstein repair. Surg Endosc 21(4):634–640, Epub 2007 Feb 16

35. Bittner R, Arregui ME, Bisgaard T, Dudai M, Ferzli GS, Fitzgibbons RJ, Fortelny RH, Klinge U, Kockerling F, Kuhry E, Kukleta J, Lomanto D, Misra MC, Montgomery A, Morales-Conde S, Reinpold W, Rosenberg J, Sauerland S, Schug-Pass C, Singh K, Timoney M, Weyhe D, Chowbey P (2011) Guidelines for laparoscopic (TAPP) and endoscopic (TEP) treatment of inguinal hernia [International Endohernia Society (IEHS)]. Surg Endosc 25:2773–2843

36. Lowham AS, Filipi CJ, Fitzgibbons RJ Jr, Stoppa R, Wantz GE, Felix EL, Crafton WB (1997) Mechanisms of hernia recurrence after preperitoneal mesh repair. Ann Surg 225:422–431

37. Felix EL, Harbertson N, Vartanian S (1999) Laparoscopic hernioplasty. Significant complications. Surg Endosc 13:328–331

38. Heikkinen T, Bringman S, Ohtonen P, Kunelius P, Haukipuro K, Hulkko A (2004) Five-year outcome of laparoscopic and Lichtenstein hernioplasties. Surg Endosc 18:518–522

39. Agrawal A, Avill R (2006) Mesh migration following repair of inguinal hernia: a case report and review of literature. Hernia 10:79–82

40. Hume RH, Bour J (1996) Mesh migration following laparoscopic inguinal hernia repair. J Laparoendosc Surg 6(5):333–335
41. Bodenbach M et al (2002) Intravesical migration of a polypropylene mesh implant 3 years after laparoscopic transperitoneal hernioplasty. Urologe A 41(4):366–368
42. Nowak DD et al (2005) Large scrotal hernia: a complicated case of mesh migration, ascites, and bowel strangulation. Hernia 9(1):96–99
43. Chuback JA et al (2000) Small bowel obstruction resulting from mesh plug migration after open inguinal hernia repair. Surgery 127(4):475–476
44. Lange B, Langer C, Markus PM, Becker H (2003) Mesh penetration of the sigmoid colon following a transabdominal preperitoneal hernia repair. Surg Endosc 17(1):157. doi:10.1007/s00464-002-4246-x
45. Rieger N, Brundell S (2002) Colovesical fistula secondary to laparoscopic transabdominal preperitoneal polypropylene (TAPP) mesh hernioplasty. Surg Endosc 16(1):218–219
46. Goswami R, Babor M, Ojo A (2007) Mesh erosion into caecum following laparoscopic repair of inguinal hernia (TAPP): a case report and literature review. J Laparoendosc Adv Surg Tech A 17:669–672
47. Ferzli GS, Frezza EE, Pecoraro AM Jr, Ahern KD (1999) Prospective randomized study of stapled versus unstapled mesh in a laparoscopic preperitoneal inguinal hernia repair. J Am Coll Surg 188(5):461–465
48. Khajanchee YS, Urbach DR, Swanstrom LL, Hansen PD (2001) Outcomes of laparoscopic herniorrhaphy without fixation of mesh to the abdominal wall. Surg Endosc 15(10):1102–1107
49. Beattie GC, Kumar S, Nixon SJ (2000) Laparoscopic total extraperitoneal hernia repair: mesh fixation is unnecessary. J Laparoendosc Adv Surg Tech A 10(2):71–73
50. Spitz JD, Arregui ME (2000) Sutureless laparoscopic extraperitoneal inguinal herniorrhaphy using reusable instruments: two hundred three repairs without recurrence. Surg Laparosc Endosc Percutan Tech 10(1):24–29
51. Ellner S, Daoud I, Gulleth Y (2006) Over five hundred laparoscopic totally extraperitoneal hernia repairs using mesh without fixation. Oral presentation (S061) at Society of American Gastrointestinal and Endoscopic Surgeons annual meeting Dallas. April 26–29
52. Moreno-Egea A, Torralba Martinez JA, Morales Cuenca G, Aguayo Albasini JL (2004) Randomized clinical trial of fixation vs nonfixation of mesh in total extraperitoneal inguinal hernioplasty. Arch Surg 139(12):1376–1379
53. Lovisetto F, Zonta S, Rota E, Mazzilli M, Bardone M, Bottero L, Faillace G, Longoni M (2007) Use of human fibrin glue (Tissucol) versus staples for mesh fixation in laparoscopic transabdominal preperitoneal hernioplasty: a prospective, randomized study. Ann Surg 245(2):222–231
54. Akolekar D, Kumar S, Khan LR, De Baux A, Nixon S (2008) Comparison of recurrence with lightweight composite polypropylene mesh and heavyweight mesh in laparoscopic totally extraperitoneal inguinal hernia repair: an audit of 1,232 repairs. Hernia 12:39–43
55. Bringman S, Blomqvist P (2005) Intestinal obstruction after inguinal and femoral hernia repair: a study of 33,275 operations during 1992–2000 in Sweden. Hernia 9:178–183 (2C)
56. Duran JJ, May JM, Msika S, Gaschard D, Domergue J, Gainant A, Fingerhut A (2000) Prevalence and mechanisms of small intestinal obstruction following laparoscopic abdominal surgery. Arch Surg 135:208–212 (2C)
57. Eugene JR, Gashti M, Curras EB, Schwartz K, Edwards J (1998) Small bowel obstruction as a complication of laparoscopic extraperitoneal inguinal hernia repair. J Am Osteopath Assoc 98:510–511 (2C)
58. Bittner R, Schmedt CG, Leibl BJ (2003) Transabdominal pre-peritoneal approach. In: LeBlanc KA (ed) Laparoscopic hernia surgery. Arnold Publisher, London, pp 54–64, 2C
59. Bittner R, Leibl BJ, Ulrich M (2006) Chirurgie der Leistenhernie. Karger, Freiburg, 2C
60. Lovisetto F, Zonta S, Rota E, Bottero L, Faillace G, Turra G, Fantini A, Longoni M (2007) Laparoscopic TAPP hernia repair: surgical phases and complications. Surg Endosc 21:646–652 (2B)

61. Lodha K, Deans A, Bhattacharya P, Underwood JW (1990) Obstructing internal hernia complicating totally extraperitoneal inguinal hernia repair. J Laparoendosc Adv Surg Tech A 8:167–168 (4)
62. McKay R (2008) Preperitoneal herniation and bowel obstruction post laparoscopic inguinal hernia repair: case report and review of the literature. Hernia 12:535–537 (4)
63. Ross SW, Oommen B, Kim M, Walters AL, Augenstein VA, Todd Heniford B (2015) Tacks, staples, or suture: method of peritoneal closure in laparoscopic transabdominal preperitoneal inguinal hernia repair effects early quality of life. Surg Endosc 29(7):1686–1693
64. Köhler G, Mayer F, Lechner M, Bittner R (2015) Small bowel obstruction after TAPP repair caused by a self-anchoring barbed suture device for peritoneal closure: case report and review of the literature. Hernia 19:389–394
65. Fitzgerald HL, Orenstein SB, Novitsky YW (2010) Small bowel obstruction owing to displaced spiral tack after laparoscopic TAPP inguinal hernia repair. Surg Laparosc Endosc Percutan Tech 20(3):e132–e135. doi:10.1097/SLE.0b013e3181dfbc05
66. Di Lorenzo N, Coscarella G, Lirosi F, Gaspari A (2002) Port-site closure: a new problem, an old device. JSLS 6:181–183
67. Yee DS, Duel BP (2006) Omental herniation through a 3-mm umbilical trocar site. J Endourol 20:133–134
68. Reardon PR, Preciado A, Scarborough T, Matthews B, Marti JL (1990) Hernia at 5-mm laparoscopic port- site presenting as early postoperative small bowel obstruction. J Laparoendosc Adv Surg Tech A 9:523–525
69. Owens M, Barry M, Janjua AZ, Winter DC (2011) A systematic review of laparoscopic port site hernias in gastrointestinal surgery. Surgeon 9(4):218–224 (2A)
70. Helgstrand F, Rosenberg J, Kehlet H, Bisgaard T (2011) Low risk of trocar site hernia repair 12 years after primary laparoscopic surgery. Surg Endosc 25:3678–3682. doi:10.1007/s00464-011-1776-0. (2A)
71. Mordecai SC, Warren OWN, Warren SJ (2012) Radially expanding laparoscopic trocar ports significantly reduce postoperative pain in all age groups. Surg Endosc 26(3):843–846. doi:10.1007/s00464-011-1963-z
72. Bhoyrul S, Payne J, Steffes B, Swanstrom L, Way LW (2000) A randomized prospective study of radially expanding trocars in laparoscopic surgery. J Gastrointest Surg 4(4):392–397 (2B)
73. Lange JFM, Kaufmann R, Wijsmuller AR, Pierie JPEN, Ploeg RJ, Chen DC, Amid PK (2014) An international consensus algorithm for management of chronic postoperative inguinal pain. Hernia. doi:10.1007/s10029-014-1292-y
74. Franneby U, Sandblom G, Nordin O et al (2006) Risk factors for long-term pain after hernia surgery. Ann Surg 244:212–219
75. Kehlet H (2008) Chronic pain after groin hernia repair. Br J Surg 95(2):135–136
76. Alfieri S, Amid PK, Campanelli G et al (2011) International guidelines for prevention and management of post-operative chronic pain following inguinal hernia surgery. Hernia 15(3):239–249
77. Chen DC, Hiatt JR, Amid PK (2013) Operative management of refractory neuropathic inguinodynia by a laparoscopic retroperitoneal approach. JAMA Surg 148(10):962–967
78. Amid PK, Chen DC (2011) Surgical treatment of chronic groin and testicular pain after laparoscopic and open preperitoneal inguinal hernia repair. J Am Coll Surg 213(4):531–536
79. Aasvang EK, Gmaehle E, Hansen JB, Gmaehle B, Forman JL, Schwarz J, Bittner R, Kehlet H (2010) Predictive risk factors for persistent postherniotomy pain. Anesthesiology 112(4):957–969
80. Fortelny RH, Petter-Puchner AH, May C, Jaksch W, Benesch T, Khakpour Z, Redl H, Glaser KS (2012) The impact of atraumatic fibrin sealant vs. staple mesh fixation in TAPP hernia repair on chronic pain and quality of life: results of a randomized controlled study. Surg Endosc 26(1):249–254
81. Singh AN, Bansal VK, Misra MC, Kumar S, Rajeshwari S, Kumar A, Sagar R (2012) Testicular functions, chronic groin pain, and quality of life after laparoscopic and open mesh repair of inguinal hernia: a prospective randomized controlled trial. Surg Endosc 26(5):1304–1317

82. Schmedt CG, Sauerland S, Bittner R (2005) Comparison of endoscopic procedures vs Lichtenstein and other open mesh techniques for inguinal hernia repair: a meta-analysis of randomized controlled trials. Surg Endosc 19:188–199
83. Aasvang E, Kehlet H (2005) Chronic postoperative pain: the case of inguinal herniorrhaphy. Br J Anaesth 95:69–76 (4)
84. Lal P, Kajla RK, Chander J, Saha R, Ramteke VK (2003) Randomized controlled study of laparoscopic total extraperitoneal versus open Lichtenstein inguinal hernia repair. Surg Endosc 17:850–856
85. Eklund A, Montgomery A, Bergkvist L, Rudberg C, Swedish Multicentre Trial of Inguinal Hernia Repair by Laparoscopy (SMIL) study group (2010) Chronic pain 5 years after randomized comparison of laparoscopic and Lichtenstein inguinal hernia repair. Br J Surg 97:600–608
86. Eker HH, Langeveld HR, Klitsie PJ, van't Riet M, Stassen LP, Weidema WF, Steyerberg EW, Lange JF, Bonjer HJ, Jeekel J (2012) Randomized clinical trial of total extraperitoneal inguinal hernioplasty vs Lichtenstein repair: a long-term follow-up study. Arch Surg 147:256–260
87. Skawran S, Weyhe D, Schmitz B, Belyaev O, Bauer KH (2011) Bilateral endoscopic total extraperitoneal (TEP) inguinal hernia repair does not induce obstructive azoospermia data of a retrospective and prospective trial. World J Surg 35(7):1643–1648
88. Hallén M, Sandblom G, Nordin P, Gunnarsson U, Kvist U, Westerdahl J (2011) Male infertility after mesh hernia repair: a prospective study. Surgery 149(2):179–184, Epub 2010 Jun 12
89. Tekatli H, Schouten N, van Dalen T, Burgmans I, Smakman N (2012) Mechanism, assessment, and incidence of male infertility after inguinal hernia surgery: a review of the preclinical and clinical literature. Am J Surg 204(4):503–509
90. Peeters E, Spiessens C, Oyen R, De Wever L, Vanderschueren D, Penninckx F, Miserez M (2010) Laparoscopic inguinal hernia repair in men with lightweight meshes may significantly impair sperm motility. Ann Surg 252:240–246
91. Peeters E, Spiessens C, Oyen R, De Wever L, Vanderschueren D, Penninckx F, Miserez M (2014) Sperm motility after laparoscopic inguinal hernia repair with lightweight meshes: 3-year follow-up of a randomised clinical trial. Hernia 18(3):361–367
92. Bischoff JM, Linderoth G, Aasvang EK, Werner MU, Kehlet H (2012) Dysejaculation after laparoscopic inguinal herniorrhaphy: a nationwide questionnaire study. Surg Endosc 26(4):979–983

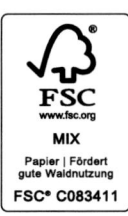

**FSC**
www.fsc.org
**MIX**
Papier | Fördert
gute Waldnutzung
**FSC® C083411**

Zeitfracht Medien GmbH
Ferdinand-Jühlke-Straße 7
99095 Erfurt, Deutschland
produktsicherheit@kolibri360.de